LABORATORY TECHNIQUES FOR HIGH SCHOOLS

A WORK-TEXT OF BIO-MEDICAL METHODS

REVISED

GABRIELLE I. EDWARDS
Assistant Principal
Supervision of Sciences
Franklin D. Roosevelt
High School
Brooklyn, New York

MARION CIMMINO
Teacher, Biology and
Laboratory Techniques
Franklin D. Roosevelt
High School
Brooklyn, New York

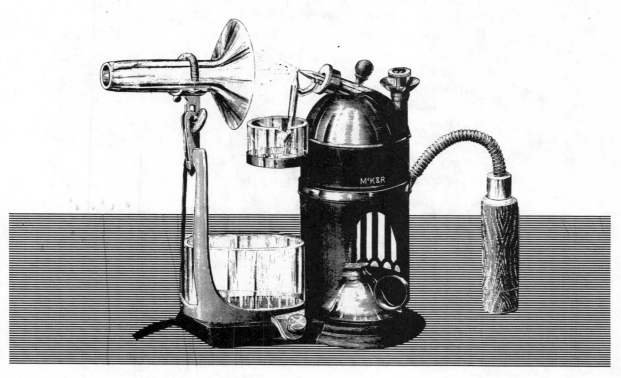

BARRON'S EDUCATIONAL SERIES, INC.   WOODBURY, NEW YORK

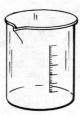

Acknowledgment

The authors wish to express their gratitude to the following companies for the use of their photographs throughout the text: Bausch and Lomb, pp. 66, 71; Beckman Instrument Company, p. 60; Corning Glass Works, p. 41; Difco Laboratories, pp. 152, 154, 161, 166, 171, 173; Ohaus Scale Corporation, p. 30.

All inquiries should be addressed to:
Barron's Educational Series, Inc.
113 Crossways Park Drive
Woodbury, New York   11797

Library of Congress Catalog Card No. 75-23111
Library of Congress Cataloging in Publication Data

Edwards, Gabrielle I
  Laboratory techniques for high schools.

  Bibliography: p.
  SUMMARY: Introduces the student to the general methods
of laboratory work and to the specialized fields of
hematology, bacteriology, and urinalysis.
  1. Biology—Laboratory manuals.   2. Medicine,
Clinical—Laboratory manuals.   [1. Biology—Laboratory
manuals.   2. Medicine, Clinical—Laboratory manuals]
I. Cimmino, Marion, joint author.   II. Title.
QH317.E38   1975   616.07'56'028   75-23111
ISBN 0-8120-0649-6 pbk.

  3 4 5 6 7 8 9 10 11   M   7 6
International Standard Book No. 0-8120-649-6

PRINTED IN THE UNITED STATES OF AMERICA

Table of Contents

To The Student

Today, there is a need for highly skilled medical laboratory assistants. This work-text has been written so that you may learn some of the basic laboratory techniques which are employed in laboratories. It is hoped that at the completion of this course, you will not only become aware of new careers open to you, but also get the feel of working in a laboratory.

You, yourself, will work through the laboratory lessons. Each laboratory lesson has been written so that you may accomplish the work in a single class period.

Since this course is a survey course, the work text has been divided into 4 units. Each unit is geared to familiarize you with some aspects of laboratory technology. Unit I, General Techniques, introduces you to the use of basic laboratory equipment. Other units in specialized areas such as bacteriology, hematology, and urinalysis will follow upon the completion of this unit.

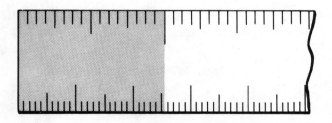

To The Teacher

Preface

In recent years emphasis has been placed upon providing a course in biology for the high school student who wishes to develop specialized laboratory skills. We, as teachers, know of the great need for trained medical and laboratory technicians. However, many students are not aware of the job opportunities in hospital and commercial laboratories. It is therefore important to expose high school students to career possibilities related to the field of biology.

The purpose of this work-text in Laboratory Techniques is to provide a *course of study* for teachers who wish to offer this course. It is applicable to students interested in medical professions (doctors, nurses, laboratory technicians, researchers) and to other students who are interested in health careers but do not plan to attend college. This course will introduce students to the specialized fields of hematology, bacteriology and urinalysis, as well as to the general methods of laboratory work.

How To Use This Book

Each lesson is divided into four parts. A simply stated *problem* delimits the scope of the lesson.

The *background information* serves as a brief introduction, explaining the purpose of the procedure and the value of the lesson. At times, the introduction may be expanded into a full period lesson in itself, depending upon the needs and ability of the class.

The next part of the lesson is the *procedure*. Each lesson has been designed so that every student can perform the required task, himself. It is advisable for the teacher to demonstrate the procedure before the students begin so that pupils can be alerted to the "dangers" or problems inherent in the lesson.

The *summary* concludes each lesson. It is composed of a series of questions based on the given lesson or the relationship between this lesson and a previous one.

Supply Check List

Your teacher may give you a numbered drawer containing the pieces of equipment listed below. Please check to be sure that all equipment listed is in good condition. At the end of the term, you will be required to return all equipment loaned to you.

RETURNABLE MATERIALS

1 slide box
10 glass slides
10 cover slips
1 glass depression slide
2 dropping bottles
1 metric ruler
1 pair of forceps
1 bunsen burner

2 beakers
1 test tube rack
5 test tubes
1 wing top
1 glass marking pencil
1 test tube holder
3 pipettes
1 wire loop
1 microscope lamp

You will be responsible for loss and breakage of the above equipment. In addition you will be required to provide the following items:

soap and soap dish
1 sponge
lab coat or apron

Safety Procedures in the Laboratory

1. Each laboratory exercise should be read before attempting to do it. Particular attention should be paid to words which are capitalized and in parenthesis.
2. No one is to begin any work without the consent of the teacher.
3. You should pay strict attention to instructions and directions before beginning an exercise.
4. Do not taste any chemicals.
5. Use caution when removing stoppers or corks from containers.
6. If you spill acid or alkali on yourself or your clothing, use plenty of water to wash them off. Report the incident to your teacher immediately.
7. If you spill chemicals on the tables, make sure to wash them off with a sponge immediately. Rinse off the sponge at once.
8. Used chemicals should not be poured back into stock bottles.
9. When lighting a burner, first remove the match from the box and then *close* the box. Strike the match and move it up along the side of the burner. Then turn on the gas.
10. Never leave a lighted burner unattended.
11. Never reach over an exposed flame.
12. Do not sit when the burner is in use.
13. Long hair must be tied back when working in the laboratory.
14. If the room is too light, draw the shades when burners are in use.
15. Always hold a test tube containing a liquid that you are heating in such a way that it will not splatter on you or your neighbor if it starts to boil.
16. Never pick up heated glass or metal with unprotected hands. Use a holder.
17. Do not leave hot pieces of equipment on the tables without warning others of their presence.
18. When working with bacteria, always wash hands thoroughly with soap and water at the end of the period.
19. Keep wash sinks free from debris.
20. Discard broken glass in ceramic crocks. Use pails for other refuse.
21. Keep the laboratory clean at all times. Make sure all equipment is cleaned and in order before leaving the laboratory.
22. All work is to stop at the teacher's five minute warning signal.
23. Report any accident to the teacher immediately.

Safety Promise

Last Name   First Name

Address

Lab.   Room   Lab. Sec.

Student's Statement

This is to certify that I have received VERBAL and PRINTED INSTRUCTIONS regarding the procedures to be followed in the laboratory. I realize that failure to observe these instructions may lead to serious consequences. Therefore, to avoid any injuries to persons or equipment, I PROMISE TO OBSERVE AND OBEY THESE RULES CAREFULLY AND FAITHFULLY.

Student's signature   Lab. Sec.   Date

Parent's signature

SPECIMEN FORM

Unit I

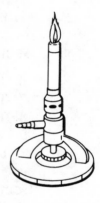

General
Techniques

Unit 1 Table of Contents

Section I

Section II

Section III

Section IV

Section V

Section VI

Section VII

Section VIII

Section IX

Problem # To identify some of the basic equipment used in the laboratory.

Background Information

Every laboratory is supplied with standard glassware which enables the technician to carry out fundamental operations. Some of the equipment has unusual names, but most have names which help you to understand their use.

Glassware in particular is vital for laboratory work. On most pieces of glassware, there are etched lines. Each line has a meaning. The lines represent a specific capacity, a certain amount of material which can be held at that level in the glassware. To indicate the capacity, a number is associated with each line. Because the etchings follow an ascending or descending numerical value, a piece of glassware which is etched is said to be graduate. Graduate glassware is used in measuring a specific amount. Glassware without gradations will be used to treat, mix, store, or process materials.

Procedure

☐ 1. Make a sketch of each piece of equipment you have received. Be sure to include as much detail as possible.

☐ 2. Identify each piece of equipment by comparing it to the pictures below.

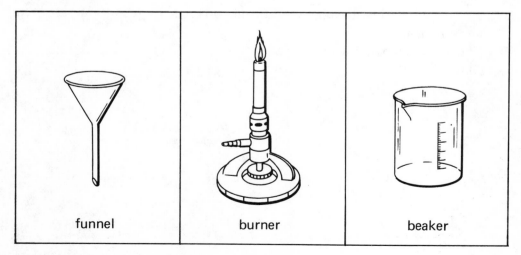

| funnel | burner | beaker |

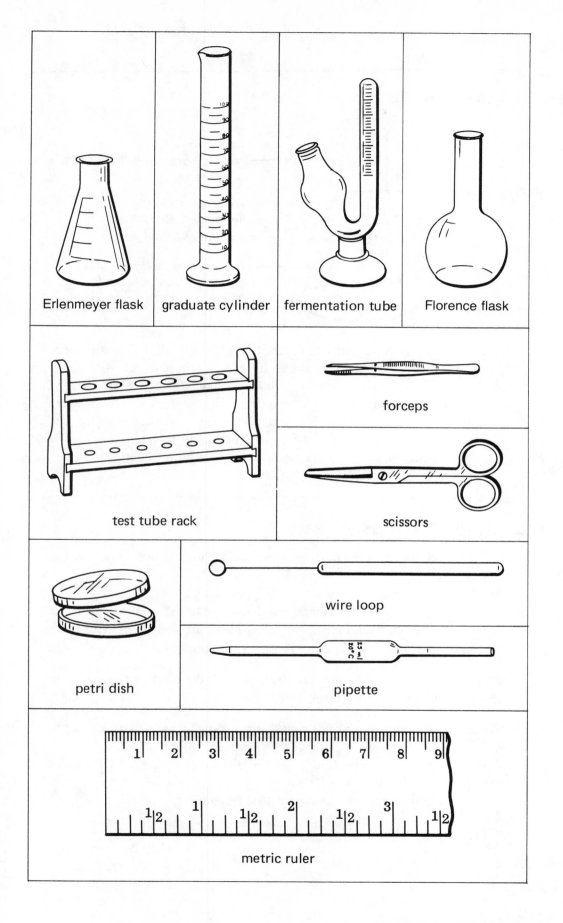

Erlenmeyer flask   graduate cylinder   fermentation tube   Florence flask

test tube rack   forceps

scissors

petri dish   wire loop

pipette

metric ruler

Lesson 1

VOLUMENTRIC GLASSWARE

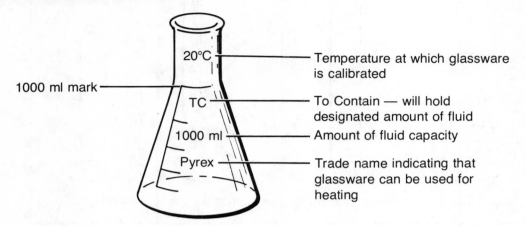

1000 ml mark

20°C — Temperature at which glassware is calibrated

TC — To Contain — will hold designated amount of fluid

1000 ml — Amount of fluid capacity

Pyrex — Trade name indicating that glassware can be used for heating

Volumetric glassware is designed to measure fluid. The markings on the piece of glassware give you information about its use. Each piece of volumetric glassware is designed to carry out a specific kind of measuring. If the piece of glassware is graduated (has graduated markings), it can be used to measure varying amounts of fluid. If there is a single level mark, as shown above, the piece of glassware is designed to measure accurately the specified amount. If glassware contains the Pyrex or Kimax label, it can be used for heating.

Questions for Review

1. List any equipment you have at your table which is not shown in this lesson.
2. What do you notice on the sides of the glassware?
3. What is the purpose of the numbers and abbreviations?
4. How are the measurements on the glassware different from the measurements that you use every day?

Study the diagrams of glassware. On the basis of these diagrams and on your knowledge, answer the questions below.

5. Which pieces of glassware can be used for heating? How do you know?
6. Which pieces of glassware can be used for measuring?
7. How can the measuring ability of the Erlenmeyer flask be extended beyond that of the Florence flask?
8. What information does the medicine glass provide?

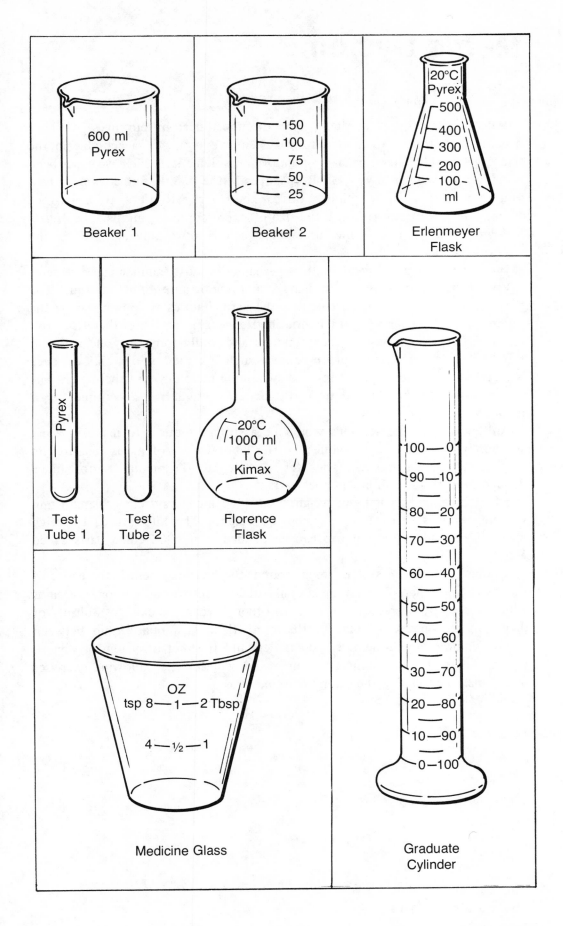

Beaker 1

Beaker 2

Erlenmeyer Flask

Test Tube 1

Test Tube 2

Florence Flask

Medicine Glass

Graduate Cylinder

Metric System

Preface

When isn't a quart a quart? For the most part of our lives, we have become accustomed to a measuring system which is not acceptable in the scientific world. The English system of measurement, which we have been using, allows you to buy a pound of grapes in the A & P, but does not allow you to prepare a prescription. You can buy a rug to fit a 10 x 12 foot room, but you cannot measure the size of microscopic organisms. The *Metric System* is the system of measurement which is universally accepted in the scientific world.

What can you measure? Length is perhaps the most familiar measurement. Everyone has used a ruler to measure something or another at one time. The most commonly used measurement is the yard. Fabrics are purchased by the square yard. There is no yard in the metric system; neither is there the foot or inch. There are, however, centimeters and millimeters. Anyone who has watched an international athletic contest, such as a race, knows that distance is measured in meters. Ski jumps and swimming races also use the meter. The meter can easily be divided into 100 or 1000 equal parts, centimeters or millimeters.

A liter of gas, please! This would be a strange request to make in a gas station. It is not a strange request in the laboratory. Volume is measured in liters in the metric system. The liter is related to the meter. It too can be divided into 1000 (milliliter) equal parts.

54.5 Kilograms! Am I overweight? Like the metric system of length and volume, there is also a metric system of weights. The kilo is used to weigh materials in this system. It too can be divided into 1000 equal parts called grams.

Strange as the new system might sound, the metric system is the easier of the two. Note that this system is easily divided into hundreds or thousands which can easily be reduced to tens. In other words, it is easy to multiply or divide in the metric system. Furthermore, there is a relationship between length, volume, and weight. If you understand the metric system of weight, you understand the system of volume and length. The following exercises will explain and clarify the metric system.

To study the metric system related to length.

Problem

Lesson 2

Background Information

You have been given a meter stick. Notice that there are two sides. On one side the measurement is in inches (English system) and on the other side the measurement is in the metric system.

The *meter* is the *fundamental* unit of measurement in the metric system. It is called the fundamental unit because it is from this standard that the metric system of weights and volume is derived.

There are 1000 equal divisions on the meter stick. The prefix milli means 1/1000. Since one part out of 1000 is called a millimeter (mm), there are 1000 mm in a meter stick.

Ten millimeters are grouped into one centimeter. The prefix centi means 1/100. There are 100 centimeters (cm) in one meter (m).

$$1 \text{ m} = 1000 \text{ mm}$$
$$1 \text{ m} = 100 \text{ cm}$$
$$10 \text{ mm} = 1 \text{ cm}$$

Procedure

☐ A. 1. Locate the mm and cm divisions on the meter stick.

☐ 2. Draw the following lines using the meter stick:

25 cm	250 mm	32 mm	8 cm
5 cm	50 mm	45 mm	3 cm

☐ 3. Convert each of the following:

50 mm =	cm	50 cm =	m
100 mm =	cm	3 cm =	mm
250 mm =	cm	400 cm =	mm
500 mm =	m	1500 cm =	mm

Lesson 2

☐ B. You have been given a metric ruler. Notice the different sets of numbers on each edge. Place this ruler against the meter stick and locate the centimeter and millimeter divisions.

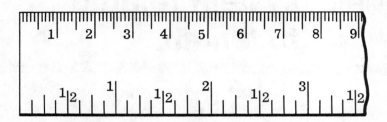

☐ 1. Convert the following:

4 in. =	cm	20 cm =	in.
6½ in. =	cm	40 cm =	in.
4½ in. =	cm	51½ cm =	in.

Questions for Review

1. What number can you multiply or divide by to solve the above problem?
2. How many cm in one foot?
3. How many mm in one foot?
4. How tall are you in feet, meters, centimeters?

Study the diagram below. Answer the questions that follow.

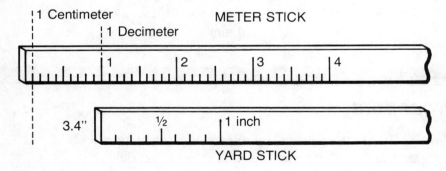

5. a) Which measuring stick is longer?
   b) By how many units is it longer?
6. a) What is the basic unit of measure of the meter stick?
   b) What is the basic unit of measure of the yard stick?
7. a) How many inches are in a yard?
   b) How many inches are in a meter?
8. Convert each of the following:
   3 yds. =   m
   5 yds. =   m
   20 yds. =   m
   58 yds. =   m

To learn the metric system related to volume.

Lesson 3

Background Information

A cube is a figure whose 6 sides are equal in length. The volume means the amount of material the cube can hold. A 10 cm cube will hold a certain amount of material. The amount of material it holds is called a *liter (l)*. The

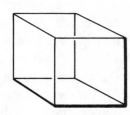

volume of the cube is measured by the length x the width x the height. The length of a 10 cm cube is 10 cm, the width is 10 cm, and the height is 10 cm. The volume is 10 cm x 10 cm x 10 cm = 1000 cc. (cc is a cubic centimeter.) Since the amount of material a 10 cm cube can hold is called a liter, 1000 cc = 1.0 *l.*

The prefix milli means 1/1000. If we divide a liter into 1000 equal parts, one part is called a millileter (ml). Therefore, 1000 ml = 1.0 *l.*

1000 ml = 1.0 *l.* = 1000 cc

Drill

☐ 1. Convert the following:

2000 cc =	*l*
4000 ml =	*l*
2500 ml =	*l*
4.0 *l* =	ml
3¼ *l* =	ml
4.0 *l* =	cc
3¼ *l* =	cc

☐ 2. How is the metric system of volume related to that of length?

☐ 3. What number is the basic unit of the metric system?

Lesson 4

To study how to use the graduate cylinder.

Background Information

One of the most useful tools in measuring volume is the graduate cylinder. Cylinder describes the shape and graduate describes the fact that there are lines equally spaced from each other. A 100 ml cylinder is most frequently used in the lab.

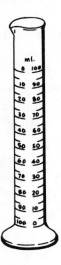

Observe that there are two sets of numbers. One set starts at zero and rises to 100 ml. The second set starts at 100 ml and rises backwards to zero. If the cylinder is filled to the top and 20 ml is to be poured out, the number on the left side is used. The liquid is poured out until the *Meniscus* reaches 20 ml. If you want to pour 20 ml into the cylinder, fill the cylinder to the 20 ml line using the right hand set of numbers. If you count the number of lines on the cylinder, there would be 100. This means that each line represents one ml. Examine cylinders of other capacities. You will note that the lines may represent some value other than one ml.

Procedure

☐ 1. Fill the cylinder with water to the 50 ml mark. Look at the water in the cylinder very carefully. You will notice that the water in the cylinder takes a special shape, bowl-like. The bottom part of the bowl is called the *MENISCUS*. The meniscus must rest on the 50 ml line. If it does not touch the 50 ml line, you will have to add or remove some water. In measuring out volume from a cylinder the meniscus must always rest on the line referring to the desired volume-MENISCUS RULE.

Rules for filling

☐ 1. Fill along one side.
☐ 2. Allow some time for drainage.

Rules for emptying

☐ 1. Pour through lip.

☐ 2. Allow some time for drainage .

☐ 3. Fill a cylinder with 62 ml of water. Hold a black card behind the cylinder, then hold a white card behind the cylinder. Did you find it easier to see the meniscus with or without the cards? Explain.

☐ 4. Practice using the meniscus rule by filling the cylinder up to the 5, 22, 59, and 75 ml marks.

☐ 5. Practice using other cylinders. Fill each up to the same marks as number 4.

Questions for Review

1. Why is the cylinder called a graduate cylinder?
2. Why must you be accurate in measuring liquids?

Look at the diagram below. Answer the questions that follow.

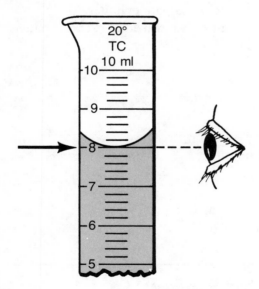

3. Define the word *meniscus.*
4. Why do we use the meniscus rule?
5. Read the level of the fluid as shown in the diagram.
6. What is the significance of the eye in the diagram?

Problem

To compare volumes in the English system to the metric system

Background Information

Review the measurement of volume in the Metric System.

$$1 \quad l. = 1000 \text{ cc or } 1000 \text{ ml}$$
$$1.0 \; l. = 1000 \text{ cc or } 1000 \text{ ml}$$

Review the use of the graduated cylinder — Meniscus rule.

Procedure

☐1. You have been given containers which hold different volumes of liquid. Fill each container with water.

☐2. Pour the water into a graduate cylinder.

☐3. Record the amount of water held in each container in ml.

☐4. Complete this chart.

English System	Metric System	
	ml	*l*
Bottle 1 fluid ounce		
4 oz.		
8 oz.		
16 oz. - 1 pt.		
32 oz. - 1 qt.		

Questions for Review

Convert the following:

1. 3 oz. to ml and *l.*
2. 1½ pt. to ml and *l.*
3. 4 qt. = 1 gallon. Convert 50 gal. to cc and *l.*
4. A 20 cm cube has a volume of 8000 cc. How many liters can it hold?

TEST YOURSELF

1. What system of measurement is used in the scientific world?
2. What is the fundamental unit of measure in this system?
3. What is the smallest division of the meter?
4. How many cm in 1 1/2 m?
5. How many ml in 1.0 *l*?
6. How many cc in 8½ *l*?
7. What rule is applied to the use of the graduate cylinder?
8. How many cm in 4 m?
9. How many mm in 4 m?
10. What is the basic multiple in the metric system?

1. _____
2. _____
3. _____
4. _____
5. _____
6. _____
7. _____
8. _____
9. _____
10. _____

Answers

1. metric
2. meter
3. mm
4. 150
5. 1000
6. 8500
7. Meniscus
8. 400
9. 4000
10. 10

To study basic
Problem **laboratory mathematic techniques.**

Background Information

All laboratory work requires the recording of numerical data. It is important to be able to read the numerical data.

Procedure

☐ 1. Reading numbers

Each number occupies a certain position.

units 1
tens 10
hundreds 100
thousands 1000
ten thousands 10000
hundred thousands 100000
millions 1000000

In the above table the number one occupies a position known as the *units* position. As one moves to the left of the units position, it changes in value. The values are indicated in the table.

Read the following numbers:

24; 91; 120; 346; 1,206; 10,451; 41,005; 101,461; 4,500,000; 6,020,401

☐ 2. Reading Decimal Numbers

There are also numbers which are less than one. These numbers are expressed as decimal numbers. Each number following a decimal occupies a special position.

.1 tenths
.01 hundredths
.001 thousandths
.0001 ten thousandths
.00001 hundred thousandths
.000001 millionths

Read the following:

.1; .02; .12; .006; .109; .2345; .021; .6; .4001; .81

☐ 3. Combine Whole and Decimal Numbers

Read the following:

1.1; 6.06; 81.29; 30.08; 100.49; 207.20; 1000.41; 1.0009; 17.101

Wherever a decimal separates two numbers, the word *and* is used in reading the numbers. The word *and* takes the place of the decimal.

☐ 4. Look at the diagrams.

Read the numbers indicated by the

a) Rain gauge
b) Stopwatch
c) Graduate cylinder

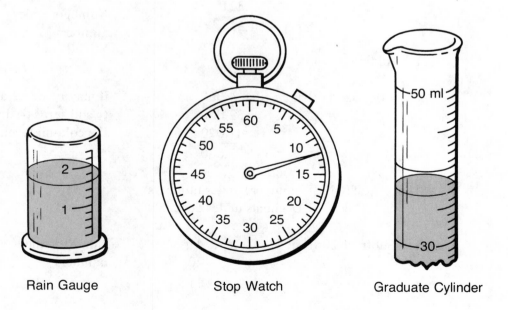

Rain Gauge   Stop Watch   Graduate Cylinder

Lesson 7

To study fundamental mathematical operations.

Background Information

In addition to being able to read basic numerical data, it is important to be able to carry out fundamental mathematical operations.

I. ADDITION – Numbers under numbers
              Decimals under decimals

a) Add

41; 6; 101	41	Numbers under
	6	numbers
	$\underline{101}$	
	148	

b) Add

.600; .410; .321	.600	Decimals under
	.410	decimals
	$\underline{.321}$	
	1.331	Numbers under
		numbers

c) Add

4.06; 32; 41.020	4.060	it may be necessary
	32.000	to add zeros to make
	$\underline{41.020}$	the columns even.
	77.080	

II. SUBTRACTION – Numbers under numbers
                 Decimals under decimals

a) Subtract 20 from 41

41	Numbers under
$\underline{-20}$	numbers
21	

b) Subtract .380 from .421

.421
−.380
.041

Decimals under decimals

c) Subtract 9.04 from 10.43

10.43
−9.04
1.39

Numbers under numbers

Decimals under decimals

III. MULTIPLICATION

24.06
x.21
2406
4812
5.0526

1. Multiply the example regardless of the presence or absence of the decimal points.
2. Count all the numbers behind the decimal points (right of points.)
3. Place the decimal point in the answer at the place corresponding to the number of decimal numbers you counted.
4. Count from right to left.

IV. DIVISION

divisor .5) 5.0 dividend

1. Move the decimal over to the end in the divisor.
2. Move the decimal over the same number of places in the dividend as in the divisor.
3. Bring the decimal to the top of the box.
4. Divide as if there was no decimal point.

.5) 5

1. Move decimal over in the divisor.

5) 5.

2. Add a decimal after the number in the dividend.

5) 5.0

3. Add as many zeros after the decimal in the dividend as the number of places in the divisor.

4. Move the decimal point in the dividend over.

5) 50.

5. Bring decimal to the top.

6. Divide.

Lesson 7

V. AVERAGES

.40; 1.60; 1.00

Add
Divide by the number of
groups that you added.

```
  .40
 1.60
 1.00
 ────
 3.00
```

```
       1.00
    ─────────
 3 ) 3.00
```

Questions for Review

Compute each of the following:

1. Addition

   a) 0.3 + 0.5 + 0.7 + 0.9

   b) .03 + .05 + .07 + .09

   c) 7.8 + 7.5 + 9.6 + 3.9

   d) .35 + 6.3 + .79 + 6.4

   e) 52 + 5.2 + 5.2 + .051

2. Multiplication

   a) 86.3 x 0.5

   b) .027 x 0.24

   c) 97.2 x 2.13

   d) 53.4 x 02.6

   e) 6.39 x 25.4

   f) 7.21 x .004

   g) .006 x 6.98

   h) 9.75 x 7.06

3. Division

   a) 29.6 ÷ 0.2

   b) 8.562 ÷ 0.3

   c) 1824 ÷ 9.6

   d) 32.66 ÷ 0.71

   e) 30.56 ÷ .08

   f) 47.7 ÷ .09

   g) 36.9 ÷ 4.1

   h) 5.562 ÷ 6.18

To learn significant digits.

Background Information

When recording data such as length, weight, volume, etc., the data should represent the greatest accuracy possible with the measuring instruments (tools) used.

Procedure

☐1. Examine your metric ruler. Find the mm divisions. Notice that you can divide the mm divisions in half. Locate the following on the ruler below: —

13.5 mm	1.5 mm
9.5	2.5
.5	3.5
10.5	4.5

Record the letter that represents your answer.

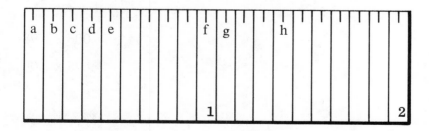

☐2. Draw the following lines:
2.5 mm, 2.05 mm, 9.15 mm, 6.55 mm, 10.05 mm.

☐3. The metric ruler can also be read in cm. Locate the following on the ruler above.

.05 cm   .45 cm
.15   1.05
.25   1.35
.35

☐4. Draw the following lines:

2.65 cm, 2.06 cm, 10.05 cm, 6.55 cm.

Questions for Review

1. What is the relationship between cm and mm?
2. In which system (English or metric) would accuracy of measurement be obtained more easily? Explain.
3. Express each of the following numbers, correct to one less signficant digit.

36.92	7.6	372.5	10.3
270.7	4.025	216.07	3492.0
21.3	19.38	10.07	17.98

To learn how to read the numbers on a triple beam balance (scale).

Lesson 9

Background Information

You have been given a triple beam balance-scale. Notice that the beam closest to you looks like your metric ruler. Each number represents a gram. Each gram in turn is divided into 10 equal parts, tenths of a gram. This beam is read like your centimeter ruler. The other beams are slightly different but can be read easily.

Procedure

☐ 1. Move the sliding rider of the beam closest to you to the following positions:

.2 g   1.2 g   3.1 g   8.9 g   10.0 g   8.5 g   .9 g   6.8 g   7.6 g
2.4 g   5.7 g   4.8 g

☐ 2. Move the second rider to the following positions:

100g   300g   500g
200g   400g

☐ 3. Move the third rider to the following positions:

10g   30g   50g   70g   90g
20g   40g   60g   80g   100g

Questions for Review

1. Into how many equal parts was the beam closest to you divided?
2. How do you read this beam?
3. What is the capacity of your scale?

Lesson 10

To learn how to operate a triple beam balance.

Background Information

You have received a single pan, triple beam balance. Notice that there is a pointer resting at zero on the right hand side. Connected to the pointer there are three beams. The beam nearest to you is divided into 10 equal parts. Each division is one gram. Each division (gram) is also sub-divided into 10 equal parts. Each of these smaller divisions is equal to a tenth of a gram. The second beam is divided into five equal parts. Each division is equal to 100 grams. The third beam is divided into 10 equal parts. Each division is equal to ten grams.

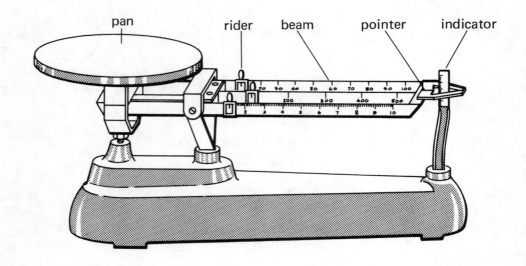

pan   rider   beam   pointer   indicator

Procedure

☐ 1. Place a small cork on the pan. Notice that the pointer rises above zero. Move the rider of the beam closest to you until the pointer rests at zero. Read the weight that the rider is pointing to. Return the rider to zero on the beam and remove the cork.

☐ 2. Place a 50 ml beaker on the pan. Notice that the pointer rises above zero. Move the rider on the first beam. If the pointer does not move from its position, the beaker is heavier than the added weight.

Move the rider on the second beam after the first has been returned to zero. If the pointer moves below zero, you have added too much weight. Continue to move the rider until you can determine the approximate weight of the beaker. If 200g is too much weight and 100g is too little weight, place the rider on the lower weight.

Move the rider on the third beam. Determine the approximate weight of the beaker. Follow the above procedure.

Move the rider on the first beam until the scale is balanced-pointer at zero.

Total the weights of the three beams. This is the weight of the beaker.

☐3. Fill the beaker with sand and re-weigh following the above procedures.

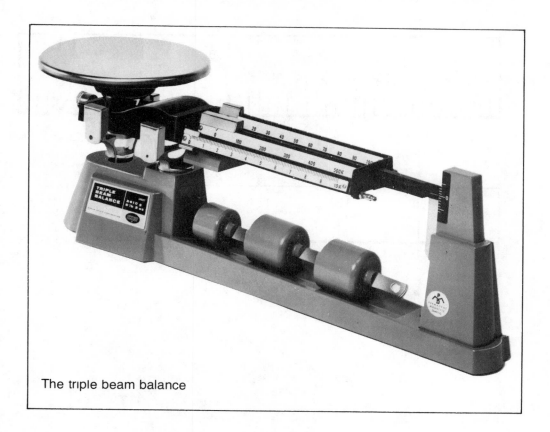

The triple beam balance

Questions for Review

1. Why do you return the rider to zero before removing the materials from the pan?

Lesson 10

2. Look at the first beam of your balance. What is the smallest amount that it can weigh accurately? What is the largest amount?
3. What is the weight range for which beam 2 is calibrated?
4. What is the smallest amount that can be weighed by beam three?
5. The scale on which you weigh yourself in the doctor's office has two beams. Let us suppose that the riders are in the following positions in response to a person's weight. How much does the individual weigh?

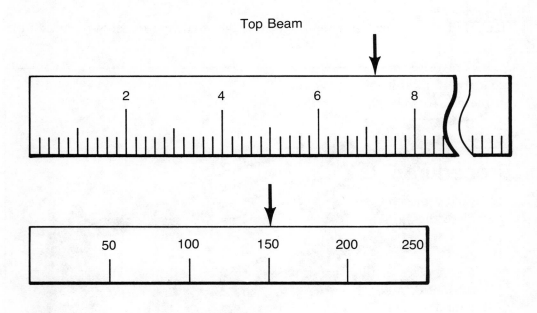

Top Beam

Lower Beam

Laboratory Techniques

Background Information

There are very few substances that can be placed directly on the pan of a scale. Corrosive or wet substances will damage the pan and decrease the accuracy of measurement. Therefore, filter paper or glassware is usually used on the pan to weigh out the substances.

Procedure

1. Fold a piece of filter paper into a small dish.
2. Place the paper on the pan and weigh.
3. Add the weight of the filter paper to the weight of the substance. Set your rider for that weight.
   Ex. A piece of filter paper weighs .6g. You wish to weigh out 2.5g of a substance. Add 2.5g to .6g = 3.1g. Set the rider to 3.1g.
4. Pour the substance into the filter paper until the pointer rests at zero. If you added too much of the substance, the pointer rises above zero. Remove the extra material with a spatular.
5. Carry out the same procedure as above for a liquid. Use a beaker, however, instead of filter paper.
6. Weigh out the following substances:

sand	water
2.7g	4.5g
15.0g	11.3g
11.9g	22.0g

Questions for Review

1. Why do you weigh the filter paper or beaker before adding a substance?
2. Why should most substances be placed on filter paper or in beakers before weighing?

Problem

To learn relationship of Metric system of weights to English system and to Metric system of volume.

Lesson 12

Background Information

When you weighed materials, you recorded the weight in grams. The gram is the basic unit in the Metric system of weights. It is related to volume in the Metric system in a very special way. In addition the gram is related to the English system of weights.

Procedure

☐ 1. Weigh a graduate cylinder.
☐ 2. Add one ml of water-use a dropper.
☐ 3. Reweigh cylinder.
☐ 4. Determine the weight of one ml of water.
☐ 5. Weigh each of the prepared containers. The labels show their weights in the English system.
☐ 6. Complete this chart.

English system	Metric system
½ lb.	
1 lb.	
3 lbs.	
5 lbs.	

Questions for Review

1. What is the relationship of the g to the ml?
2. How much does 1 ml of water weigh?
3. How much does 1 *l* of water weigh?
4. How much do you weigh in the Metric system?
5. Convert

2 oz = _____ g   350 cc = _____ g
1-1/2 lb = _____ g   680 ml = _____ g
4 lb = _____ g

Background Information

The triple beam balance enabled you to weigh materials with .1g (tenth) accuracy. Most materials must be weighed with more accuracy, especially pharmaceutical products. The Dial-O-Gram scale gives us .01g (hundredths) accuracy.

The scale consists of a beam with a 100g capacity. There is also a dial and a vernier. The dial is divided into 10 g. Each gram is sub-divided into 10 equal parts. Each line on the dial is equal to .1g. The dial is read like the first beam of the triple beam balance. The vernier divides each .1g into ten equal parts. Each line on the vernier is equal to .01g.

Procedure

☐1. Place the cork to be weighed on the pan.
☐2. The pan is unlocked.
☐3. The rider on the beam is moved.
☐4. The dial is turned SLOWLY until the scale is balanced.
☐5. The pan is locked.
☐6. Read the total weights.
☐7. Remove the substance from the pan and return the rider and dial to zero.

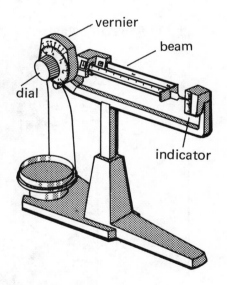

How to Read the Dial

☐1. Read the number on the dial that is opposite to the zero of the vernier.
☐2. You may notice that the zero line of the vernier is between lines on the dial.
☐3. Read the dial to the nearest tenth.

Lesson 13

□ 4. Look on the vernier to find another line that matches up with a line on the dial.

□ 5. Read the hundredths number on the vernier.

□ 6. Add the weights of the beam, dial, and vernier.

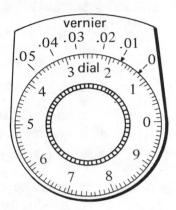

Example
$$A = 1.2 \quad \text{(dial)}$$
$$B = \underline{\;\;.01\;\;} \quad \text{(vernier)}$$
$$\text{total} \quad 1.11$$

Questions for Review

1. What part of the scale is similar to the first beam in the triple beam balance?

2. Why must the pan be locked before loading and unloading materials?

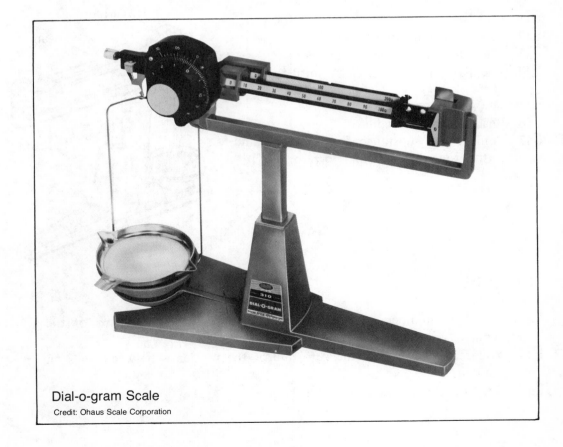

Dial-o-gram Scale

Problem To learn how to operate the double pan balance.

Procedure

☐ 1. Observe the swing of the needle. If it swings evenly on both sides, the scale is balanced. If the swing is uneven, adjust by turning the wheel in the proper direction.

☐ 2. Place an object on the left pan (convention).

☐ 3. Observe the swing of the needle.

☐ 4. In order to balance the scale, weights must be added to the right pan. *Handle weights with forceps only*.

☐ 5. Weigh each piece of equipment at your desk except the pipettes. Record.

☐ 6. Weigh each lettered empty bottle. Record.

☐ 7. Fill each lettered bottle to capacity with water. Weigh and record.

☐ 8. Fill a bottle with the following amounts of water:

23 ml, 50 ml, 61 ml, 103 ml, 210 ml.

Weigh and record the weight of the *water* only.

☐ 9. Weigh out the following amounts of sand in a beaker:

5g, 24g, 39g, 110g.

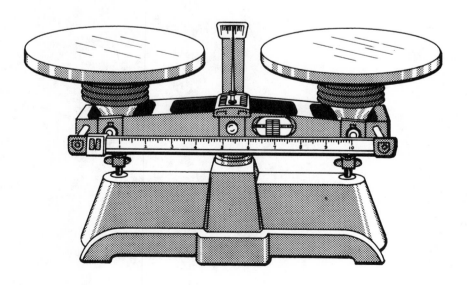

Lesson 14

☐ 10. Complete this chart.

desk equipment	weight
empty bottle A B C D	weight
lettered bottle plus 23 ml 50 ml 61 ml 103 ml 210 ml	weight

Questions for Review

1. Why are forceps used to handle the weights?
2. How many parts to a gram?
3. How does the accuracy of this scale compare to the accuracy of the triple beam balance?

To learn how to use the Dietary Scale.

Procedure

☐ 1. Under the platform there is a small knob. In order to line the needle of the scale on the face with zero, this knob can be turned.

☐ 2. Observe the face of the scale. The gradations are in multiples of 10. Each 10 g is further divided into 5 parts. Each gradation equals 2 g. The capacity of this scale is the value shown on the face, 500g.

☐ 3. On the side of the face of the scale, there is a handle. This handle turns a disc that looks exactly like the values on the face.

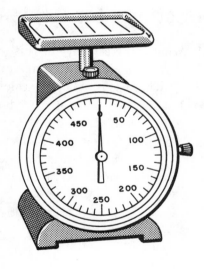

☐ 4. The capacity of the scale can be increased. Place a bottle on the platform. Turn the handle so that the zero on the disc lines up with the weight on the scale. You have changed the zero position on the scale.

☐ 5. Fill the bottle half way with water. Now, read the value from the disc not the face.

☐ 6. Fill each of the lettered bottles with the following amount of water:

30ml, 70ml, 240ml, 322ml, 444ml, 500ml, 540ml.

Record the weight of the water.

☐ 7. Weigh out the following amount of sand in a beaker:

20g, 54g, 300g, 428g, 502g

Lesson 15

☐ 8. Complete this chart.

	weight
Bottle A	
B	
C	
D	
water 30 ml	
70 ml	
240 ml	
322 ml	
444 ml	
500 ml	
540 ml	

Questions for Review

1. What is the capacity of this scale?
2. How does this scale compare in accuracy with other scales used?
3. Of what use is a dietary scale in your home?
4. Let us suppose that a wedge of cheese weighs 56.6 grams. How many ounces is this? Consult the appendix for help in conversion.
5. You were asked to weigh various volumes of water on the dietary scale. What is the relationship between volume and weight of water? The answer is contained in the diagram below.

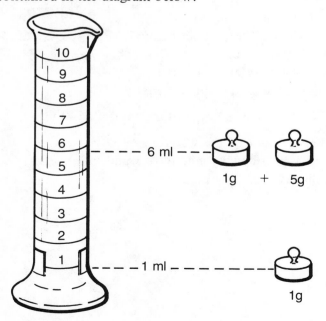

Analytical Balance

Background Information

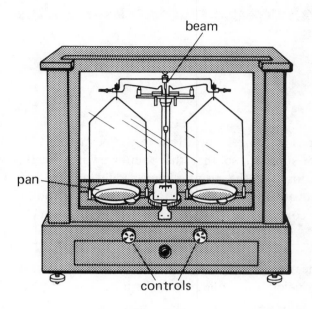

beam

pan

controls

The triple beam balance enabled you to measure the weight of objects with precision to the 0.1g while the dial-o-gram provided 0.01g accuracy. The analytical balance is a sensitive and precise instrument which allows you to measure the weight of objects with precision to the 0.1 mg or 0.0001g.

There is a horizontal beam with two pans suspended from the ends. The beam pivots (turns) about its midpoint where there is a knife edge resting against a flat surface. This contact point about which the beam turns is one of the most delicate parts of the balance and must be treated with care to prevent permanent and costly damage. Similar delicate points are found where the pans hang from the beam. To prevent damage to the three contact points the BEAMS AND PANS ARE LOCKED AT ALL TIMES; WHEN ADDING OR REMOVING WEIGHTS, WHEN OPENING OR CLOSING THE CASE, AND WHEN STORING THE BALANCE.

The beam support is controlled by a knob extending from the center of the floor of the case. The pan support is often controlled by a knob next to the beam-support control although the same knob may operate both. There is a long pointer attached to the beam and extending to a ruled scale. The deflection of the pointer enables you to see if the pans are balanced.

There is also a rider, which is operated by a hook fastened to the roof, that protrudes from the top of the case. This rider enables you to add weight in .1 mg units.

Each balance is provided with its own box of weights. The larger weights are cylindrical in shape and the smaller weights are flat pieces of metal.

Problem To learn how to operate an analytical balance.

Procedure

☐ 1. Check to see that the rider is at the zero position on the beam.

☐ 2. Release the pan and beam supports so that the pointer swings freely. Note the number of divisions that the pointer moves right and left of center. Locate the mid-point of the swing. This is the *rest point,* the point where the pointer would come to rest when the scale is in balance. Record the rest point.

☐ 3. Lock the beam and pans.

☐ 4. Open the case and place the object to be weighed in the center of the *left* pan. If the substance is a non-corrosive solid, it may be placed directly on the pan; if not, place it in a container.

☐ 5. Using forceps, put a weight which you estimate equals the weight of the object, in the right pan.

☐ 6. Close the door of the balance.

☐ 7. Release beams and pans.

☐ 8. If the pointer swings left, the weight is too heavy.

☐ 9. Lock beams and pans.

☐ 10. Remove the weight and replace with a smaller weight.

☐ 11. Close door and release beams and pans.

☐ 12. If the beam swings right, the weight is too small.

☐ 13. You will have to add weights from the beam above the pans by using the rider.

☐ 14. When the pans are balanced, lock the beams and pans. Total the weights on the pan and on the beam.

☐ 15. Remove the weights and substance from the pans and close case.

Questions for Review

1. Why are the beams and pans locked when adding or removing substances and weights from the pans?
2. Why are weights handled with forceps?
3. Why must the door be closed when using the balance?

Lesson 16

TEST YOURSELF

1. What is the beam capacity of the triple beam balance?

1. _____

2. Which scale is most sensitive?

2. _____

3. What is the accuracy of the dial-o-gram?

3. _____

4. What is the weight of 1 ml of water?

4. _____

5. How many grams are there in 1 lb?

5. _____

6. Total the following: .7, 1.4, .030

6. _____

7. Which is largest? .7, .07, .007

7. _____

8. Multiply .79 by .03

8. _____

9. What is the accuracy of the analytical balance?

9. _____

10. How many mg are there in 20 g?

10. _____

11. a) Divide 3.5868 by .84
    b)   3.5868 by 2.84

11 a. _____
    b. _____

12. How many inches are in one meter?

12. _____

13. How many decimeters are in one meter?

13. _____

14. The vernier on the Dial-o-gram scale reads accurately to which decimal?

14. _____

15. What name is given to glassware in which fluid can be measured?

15. _____

16. Of all the balances that you have used in class, which is the most sensitive?

16. _____

17. Convert 4 tablespoons to ounces.

17. _____

18. For what does the abbreviation *l* stand?

18. _____

19. 1 ml is equal to how many cc?

19. _____

20. How should metal weights be handled?

20. _____

1. 610g
2. analytical balance
3. .01g
4. 1g
5. 454g
6. 2.13
7. .7
8. .0237
9. .0001g
10. 20000 mg
11. a 4.27   b 1.26
12. 39
13. 10
14. hundredths
15. volumetric
16. analytical
17. 2 ounces
18. liter
19. 1
20. with forceps

Problem # To learn how to use a pipette.

Background Information

A pipette resembles a drinking straw. It may be filled in nearly the same way. When you place a straw in a liquid, the liquid rises slightly. The air pressure above the column of the liquid keeps it from rising all the way. If you remove the pressure, the liquid rises. The pressure may be decreased by drawing the air out of the straw. This is accomplished when you place the straw in your mouth and draw on it.

There are several types of pipettes. A pipette used for measuring a fixed volume is called a *transfer* pipette. A pipette used for measuring varying volumes is called a *graduate* pipette.

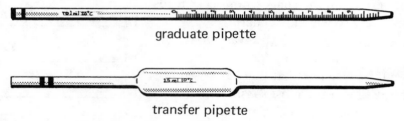

graduate pipette

transfer pipette

The pipette works on the same principle as a straw. Since it is used for accurate analysis of liquids, special care and handling must be learned.

Procedure

Filling a pipette

☐ 1. Draw the liquid above the mark you desire. (If you need 5 ml, fill it above 5 ml.)
☐ 2. Place your index finger over the open end after you have drawn the liquid up.
☐ 3. Remove the pipette from the liquid and wipe the tip.
☐ 4. Hold the pipette straight up and allow the extra liquid to run out very SLOWLY.
☐ 5. When the MENISCUS is reached, wipe the tip.

Discharging a pipette

☐ 1. By removing the index finger or applying different amounts of pressure, the liquid will flow out.
☐ 2. The liquid should flow out a drop at a time. The faster the liquid flows, the more is left behind in the tube.
☐ 3. When using a small pipette, the tip should be allowed to touch the side of the glass receiving the liquid and left in a straight position for 5 seconds. The drop at the tip is blown out.

Practice

☐ 1. Place the pipettes on the table.
☐ 2. Examine the graduate pipettes.
☐ 3. Draw each pipette.
☐ 4. Determine the capacity of each pipette.
☐ 5. Determine the value of each gradation.
☐ 6. Fill and discharge each pipette with water. Learn to control the flow of liquids in and out of the pipettes.
☐ 7. Practice drawing and delivering different amounts of water.
☐ 8. Fill and discharge the transfer pipettes.

Questions for Review

1. Why is the meniscus rule used?
2. What did you notice in filling the different sized pipettes?
3. Why is so much care taken in filling and discharging a pipette?
4. You have to measure 5.5 ml of water. What kind of pipette would you select for this job?
5. Compare the use of the graduate pipette and the delivery pipette.
6. Can you explain why water rises in a pipette?

To compare the accuracy of the pipette to the graduate cylinder - Part I.

Problem

Background Information

You have learned how to use a graduate cylinder and a pipette. Since both are used to measure volume, one must have a greater accuracy than the other.

Procedure

☐ 1. Review the use of the triple beam balance.
☐ 2. Review the meniscus rule.
☐ 3. Review the use of the graduate cylinder.
☐ 4. (a) Place a 50 ml beaker on the pan of the scale. Weigh the beaker.
    (b) Add 5 ml of water to a graduate cylinder. Empty the cylinder of water into the beaker.
    (c) Weigh the 5 ml of water. Subtract the weight of the empty beaker from the weight of the beaker and 5 ml of water. The remainder is the weight of the 5 ml of water. Record the results in the proper space on the chart.
☐ 5. Add 5 ml of water to the graduate cyliner. Empty the cylinder into the beaker on the scale. Re-weigh. Subtract the weight of the beaker and water of line 1 from line 2. The remainder is the weight of 5 ml of water.
☐ 6. Add 5 ml of water to the graduate cylinder. Empty into the beaker. Re-weigh. Subtract the weight of the beaker and water of line 2 from line 3. The remainder is the weight of 5 ml of water.
☐ 7. Total column C and average.

	A Wt of the beaker	B Wt of beaker and water	C Wt of 5 ml of water
1			
2	same		
3	same		

total _____

average _____

Questions for Review

1. What'should 5 ml of water weigh? Why?
2. Why do you not empty out the beaker before you add more water to it?
3. Why did you get a slightly different answer for the three different weighings of the water?
4. Why is the average weight the one used?

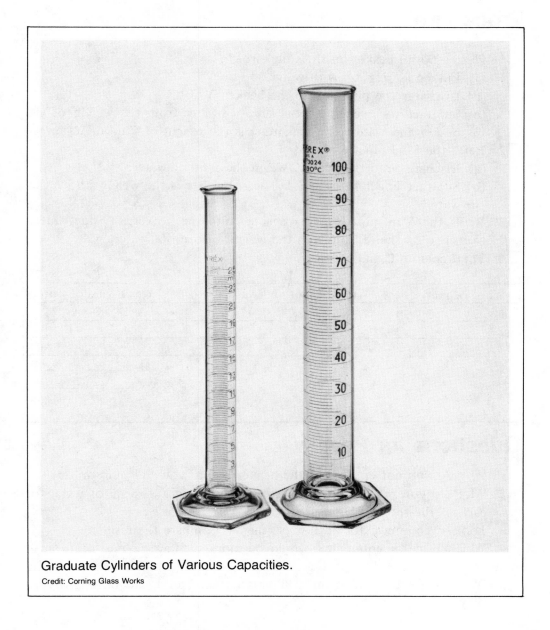

Graduate Cylinders of Various Capacities.
Credit: Corning Glass Works

Problem To compare the accuracy of the pipette to the graduate cylinder - Part II.

Procedure

☐ 1. Place a 50 ml beaker on the scale. Weigh.
 (a) Fill a 5 ml pipette with water.
 (b) Discharge the pipette into the beaker. Weigh.
 (c) Subtract the weight of the empty beaker from the weight of the beaker and water. The remainder is the weight of 5 ml of water.

☐ 2. Refill the 5 ml pipette.
 (a) Discharge into the beaker. Weigh the 5 ml of water.
 (b) Subtract line 1 from line 2. The remainder is the weight of 5 ml of water.

☐ 3. Refill the 5 ml pipette and discharge into the beaker. Subtract line 2 from line 3. The remainder is the weight of 5 ml of water.

☐ 4. Total column C and average.

	A	B	C
	Wt of beaker	Wt of beaker and water	Wt of 5 ml of water
1			
2			
3			

total _____

average_____

Questions for Review

1. Why do you not empty out the beaker before you add more water?
2. Why did you get a different answer for the weight of 5 ml of water for each of the three weighings?
3. Look at column C for both experiments. Compare the results.
4. Which piece of equipment would be more accurate in measuring small amounts of liquid?
5. Which piece of equipment will you use in blood and urine analysis? Why?

To learn how to use Problem a Bunsen burner or a Fisher burner.

Background Information

The Bunsen burner functions to mix gas with air so that a flame with a very high temperature and without soot is produced. Examine your burner and compare it to the diagram. There are two kinds of flame possible with your burner, a blue flame and a yellow flame. The color depends on the amount of air which enters. To control the amount of entering air, the collar can be turned. If the collar is closed, the flame is yellow (lack of air). A yellow flame is a cold, sooty flame. A wheel at the base of the burner controls the height of the flame.

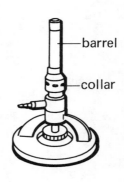

The Fisher burner has no collar. The air entrance is controlled by a lever on the under side of the burner. This lever is located in the same position as the wheel on the Bunsen burner. Except for these differences, the burner works on the same principle as the Bunsen burner.

Procedure

I. How to light the burner.

☐   1. Insert the rubber tube coming from the burner into the gas jet at your table.

☐   2. Remove a match from a box.

☐   3. Close the box of matches.

☐   4. Strike the match and bring it to the burner along the side of the barrel.

☐   5. Turn the gas jet on. The burner should light. THE FLAME FROM THE BURNER IS VERY DIFFICULT TO SEE, IF THE ROOM IS LIGHT. NEVER LEAN OVER THE BURNER. TELL YOUR NEIGHBOR THAT YOU HAVE LIT THE BURNER. NEVER SIT WHEN THE BURNER IS LIT.

II. How to adjust the burner.

☐   1. Turn the collar until you shut off the air. Notice the color of the flame.

Lesson 20

☐   2.   Hold a piece of glass in the flame for a few seconds and notice the deposit of soot at the tip.

☐   3.   Open the collar until you have a blue flame.

III. Parts of a flame.

☐   1.   You should notice that there are two parts to the blue flame, the outer and inner cone. The hottest part of this flame is at the tip of the inner cone. When you heat something, it should be held at this point.

IV. Turn off the burner.

☐   1.   Place a straight pin through the center of a match. See diagram.

☐   2.   Rest the pin across the mouth of the barrel, so that the head of the match points upward.

☐   3.   Light the burner.

☐   4.   What do you notice? How do you explain this?

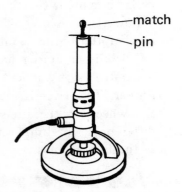

Questions for Review

1. Why does it take longer to cook something over a yellow flame?
2. What is the cause of a yellow flame in the Bunsen burner?
3. In your own words tell the differences in the flames shown below.

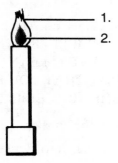

   Laboratory Techniques

To learn special glass processing techniques.

Background Information

It is often necessary to prepare very simple glass equipment. It is also necessary to know how to make a rough edged piece of glass safe for handling.

Procedure

   I. Glass Cutting

☐   1. Place the glass tubing flat on the surface of the table. With the edge of a triangular file, make a deep scratch where it is to be cut.

☐   2. Take the glass in both hands, thumb opposite the cut and ¼ inch apart.

☐   3. Apply outward pressure with your thumbs.

☐   4. If the glass is very thick, make a scratch which goes around the tube. Follow above rules.

  II. Flanging

☐   1. The purpose of flanging a tube is to finish and strengthen the ends.

☐   2. Heat the end by rotating it in the flame until it gets soft.

☐   3. Press the heated end down against an asbestos board.

III. Glass Bending

☐   1. On an asbestos board, draw the angle or shape desired.

☐   2. Place a wing top on the burner. Light the burner.

☐   3. Hold the glass in your hand so that the center of the glass is over the flame. Slowly turn the glass so that all sides are equally heated.

☐   4. When the glass is red-hot and begins to sag, remove it from the flame. Place it on the asbestos board and bend it to the desired shape. Hold it there until it hardens. A good bend has the same size in the bend as in the straight part of the tube.
CAUTION: YOU CAN GET A PAINFUL BURN FROM HOT GLASS.
BE CAREFUL – FOLLOW THE RULES.

Lesson 21

IV. Fire Polishing

☐ Broken or chipped ends may be made smooth by heating and rotating the end until the sharp edges are round.

V. Exercise

☐ 1. Cut a glass rod in half and fire polish.

☐ 2. Cut a glass tube in half. Make a right angle bend in one half. With the other half make a micro-pipette by drawing out the heated glass.

To combine the use of the scale, cylinder, and burner.

Background Information

This lesson has been designed to allow you to practice some of the skills that you have learned.

Procedure

☐ 1. Weigh 84 ml of water in a graduate cylinder.
☐ 2. Weigh an empty beaker and record its weight.
☐ 3. Weigh 4.8 g of salt and add it to the cylinder.
☐ 4. Light a burner.
☐ 5. Pour the salt solution into a test tube until it is ¼ filled.
☐ 6. Heat the test tube for one minute, paying attention to the rules below:

RULES FOR HEATING TEST TUBES

(a) Always use a test tube holder when holding a test tube in a flame.
(b) Point the test tube in such a direction so that it does not face anyone.
(c) Gently rotate the test tube as you heat it.
(d) If the material boils up to the top, remove the tube from the flame until it returns to the bottom. Then continue to heat.
(e) Always stand the heated test tube in a wooden rack.

☐ 7. After one minute, pour heated salt solution into the beaker.
☐ 8. Repeat the above exercise until all the solution has been heated at least once.
☐ 9. Weigh the contents in the beaker.
         How much does the heated solution weigh?
         What accounts for the difference in weight between the first solution and the heated solution?

Lesson 22

Questions for Review

1. Why is this exercise important?
2. Why must the test tube be held away from everyone?
3. Why do you rotate the test tube while heating it?

To study the characteristics of a solution.

Background Information

If you add salt or sugar to water, it dissolves. There are many substances which dissolve in water or alcohol. A substance which dissolves in either water or alcohol forms a solution. A *solution*, therefore, is a permanent mixture of one substance dissolved in another. The substance which dissolves is called the *solute* while the liquid in which something dissolves is called the *solvent*. Water and alcohol are two of the most common solvents; however, there are other solvents. Since you will be using many solutions in the laboratory, it is important to know some of their characteristics.

Procedure

☐ 1. Examine the 2 bottles labelled "solution."

☐ 2. Describe their colors.

☐ 3. Hold your hand behind each. Describe what you notice.

☐ 4. Examine the bottom of each bottle. Compare them to a bottle labelled "suspension." What do you notice?

☐ 5. Try to remove the solute from each solution by filtration.
   (a) Fold a piece of filter paper in half.
   (b) Fold it in half again so that there are 4 equal parts.
   (c) Turn the opened paper over. Fold one of the ¼ in half. There are now six parts.
   (d) Make another fold at right angles to the previous fold. There are now eight parts.
   (e) Divide one of the 8 parts in half.
   (f) Make a fold cutting this new area in half.
   (g) When you pick up the paper and place it in a funnel, there are 4 sides, two with a triple thickness.
   (h) Pour the contents of a solution into the funnel. The filtrate is caught in a beaker under the funnel.

☐ 6. After you have filtered the solution, examine the filter paper to see if you caught any of the solute. What is the size of the solute in a solution?

☐ 7. Filter the suspension and compare to the solution.

Lesson 23

☐ 8. Complete this chart.

Characteristic	solution	suspension
appearance (clear or cloudy)		
sedimentation		
size of solute		
distribution of solute		

Questions for Review

1. What are the characteristics of a solution?
2. How can you determine the size and distribution of the solute in a solution?

To learn how to prepare percentage solutions.

Background Information

A laboratory technician will work with solutions of different strengths. The strength of a solution may be measured by the amount of solute in an equal volume of solvent. A 90% salt solution is stronger than a 10% solution. This means that there is more solute in the 90% solution than in the 10% solution. When concentrations (strength) are measured in terms of the amount of solute in 100 cc of solvent, the solution is called a *percentage solution*. A technician must be able to prepare percentage solutions.

Procedure

   I.   Prepare an 8.5% salt solution.

- [ ]   1. Weigh 8.5g of salt.
- [ ]   2. Place salt in a large beaker. Add 50 ml of distilled water, stir until dissolved.
- [ ]   3. Pour into volumetric flask (100 ml flask).
- [ ]   4. Wash the beaker with 10 ml of distilled water and pour into flask.
- [ ]   5. Repeat step 4.
- [ ]   6. To the flask add enough distilled water to reach the 100 ml gradation.
- [ ]   7. Pour solution into stoppered bottle and label and date.

  II. Prepare a 2.5% sugar solution.

- [ ]   1. Weigh 2.5 g of sugar, place in large beaker.
- [ ]   2. Add 50 ml of distilled water, stir, pour into volumetric flask.
- [ ]   3. Wash beaker with 10 ml of water and pour into flask.
- [ ]   4. Repeat step 3.
- [ ]   5. To the flask add enough water to reach the 100 ml gradation.
- [ ]   6. Pour solution into stoppered bottle, label, and date.

 III. Prepare an 0.85% solution from the 8.5% solution.

- [ ]   1. Draw 10 ml of the 8.5% solution with a pipette.
- [ ]   2. Discharge into 100 ml flask.
- [ ]   3. Fill flask with water up to the 100 ml gradation.

Lesson 24

IV. Prepare an 0.4% 400 ml solution of salt.

☐   1.   If 0.4 g are needed for a 100 ml solution, then 1.6 g are needed for a 400 ml solution (four times as much).

☐   2.   Weigh out 1.6 g of salt.

      3.   Dissolve the solute in a large beaker to which 50 ml of water has been added. Pour into flask.

☐   4.   Wash the beaker with 10 ml of water, pour into flask.

☐   5.   Repeat step 4.

☐   6.   Fill flask up to the 400 ml gradation.

Questions for Review

1. How many grams of sugar are needed to make a 75% solution?
2. How much salt is needed to make 250 ml of a 1% solution?
3. How much boric acid is needed to prepare 500 ml of a 5% solution?
4. How would you prepare a 7.5% salt solution from the 75% solution?

GENERAL TECHNIQUES

TEST YOURSELF

1. What color should a hot flame appear?

    1. _____

2. What part of the flame of a burner is the hottest?

    2. _____

3. What do we call the process of heating glass edges to make them safe for use?

    3. _____

4. What is used to spread the flame of a burner?

    4. _____

5. What is a mixture of a solute and a solvent called?

    5. _____

6. How much salt is needed to make a 10% percentage solution?

    6. _____

7. What is one common solvent?

    7. _____

8. What type of pipette is used to measure specific amounts of a liquid?

    8. _____

9. Which is more accurate — a pipette or a graduate cylinder?

    9. _____

10. What is the dissolving agent in a solution called?

    10. _____

Answers

1. blue   2. inner cone   3. fire polishing   4. wing top   5. solution   6. 10 g   7. water   8. graduate   9. pipette   10. solvent

General Techniques
pH

When certain substances are dissolved in water, they tend to break up (dissociate) into invisible electrically charged particles. These particles are called *ions*. When an acid dissociates, hydrogen ions (H^+) are released while hydroxyl ions (OH^-) are released when a base dissociates. Every substance which dissociates does not release the same number of ions. The concentration of ions present is measured in terms of *pH*.

When water dissociates, there is an equal number of H^+ and OH^-. $H_2O \longrightarrow H^+ + OH^-$. The definition of pH is the negative log of the hydrogen ion concentration or pH = -log (H^+). With some simple logarithmic mathematics, the pH of H^+ is calculated at 7 and the pH of OH^- is also calculated at 7. If there are as many H^+ as OH^- the solution is neutral and the pH is 7. The more H^+ present, the lower the pH. The more OH^- the higher the pH.

A substance which releases H^+ is called an *acid* while a substance which releases OH^- is called a *base*. The acids or bases may be strong or weak depending on the number of ions they release. The scale below demonstrates this point.

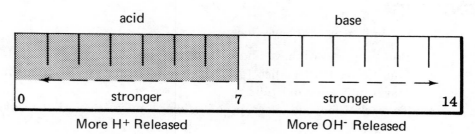

To determine the pH, *indicators* are used. Indicators are liquids or specially treated papers. They turn colors in the presence of acids or bases. Some indicators are so sensitive that they detect only a narrow range of pH while others merely detect the presence or absence of the ions.

Why fuss over the pH of a substance? All body fluids such as blood and urine have a certain normal pH. Any change in the pH indicates a disorder which may result in death. Microscopic organisms such as bacteria require a certain pH in order to grow. Different plants and trees require specific pH's in order to grow. Even tropical fish can survive in their fish tank only if the pH is correct. In general, all living organisms require a specific internal or external pH for their survival.

Problem To learn how to use liquid and paper indicators.

Background Information

Some natural food stuffs can be used as indicators. However, in the laboratory commercially prepared indicators are available. Indicators may be divided into two groups, those that indicate the specific pH of a substance and those that merely indicate if the substance is an acid or a base. Cabbage juice, litmus paper, and phenopthalein fall into the second group while Hydrion paper and Universal indicators fall into the first group.

Procedure

I. Natural indicator - cabbage juice.

☐ 1. Boil some red cabbage and collect the juice.
☐ 2. Pour some lemon juice (acid) into a test tube and baking soda (base) into a second tube.
☐ 3. To each tube add 5 drops of cabbage juice. Record the color change.
☐ 4. Continue the above procedure with each substance found on the chart. Record all color changes.

II. Phenopthalein.

☐ 1. Place 5 drops of phenolpthalein in a test tube.
☐ 2. Add 3 drops of lemon juice. Record color change.
☐ 3. Continue the above procedure until all the substances have been tested. *Make sure that each test tube is well cleaned before re-use.*

III. Litmus Paper.

☐ 1. Spread sheets of pink and blue paper on paper toweling.
☐ 2. With a stirring rod that has been dipped into lemon juice, touch the tip of each colored strip. Record color changes.
☐ 3. Continue above procedure until all substances have been tested. *Clean the rod well after each application.*

IV. Hydrion Paper - You will notice that there is a color chart with each vial of the paper. Associated with each color is a specific pH.

☐   1. Spread sheets of hydrion paper on paper toweling.

☐   2. With a stirring rod dipped in lemon juice, touch the tip of a sheet of hydrion paper.

☐   3. Compare the color of the paper to the color chart on the vial. Record.

☐   4. Continue the above procedure until all the substances have been tested.

V. Universal Indicator - This is a liquid very similar to the hydrion paper. There is a color chart with each bottle.

☐   1. Place 5 drops of lemon juice into a test tube.

☐   2. Add 5 drops of the indicator.

☐   3. Compare the color with the chart on the bottle. Record.

☐   4. Continue the above procedure until all the substances have been tested.

Substance	Cabbage juice	Phenolpthalein	Litmus paper	Hydrion paper	Universal indicator
lemon juice citric acid					
vinegar acetic acid					
HCl hydrochloric					
lye (NaOH)					
limewater Ca (OH)$_2$					
baking soda					
Mg (OH)$_2$					

Lesson 25

Questions for Review

1. Which indicator would not be used in a laboratory?
2. When litmus paper is used, which one turns color in the presence of an acid?
3. If phenolpthalein turns color, is the substance an acid or a base?
4. Which indicators give the strength of the acid or base?
5. Which is the strongest acid and base in this lesson?
6. What is the value of this lesson?

To learn how to use a Comparative Color Block Indicator.

Background Information

In addition to hydrion paper and universal indicators, there is another method for determining pH, the Comparative Color Block Indicator. A series of differently colored test tubes (standards) are provided with a plastic block, in which there are 6 transparent slots. Each color represents a specific pH. The pH is clearly marked on each tube. If a substance matches the color of one of the standards, after an indicator has been added to it, then it has the same pH of that standard. This method of determining pH is similar to a method used in determining hemoglobin content of the blood which will be learned in another unit.

Procedure

☐ 1. Fill a blank tube (that comes with the kit) with lemon juice up to the gradation line.

☐ 2. Add 5 drops of the standard indicator.

☐ 3. Stir gently to mix.

☐ 4. Place 3 distilled water tubes in the block. Use the slots closest to the plastic.

☐ 5. Place the lemon juice in a center slot of the block.

☐ 6. Choose the standards that seem to match the color of the juice.

☐ 7. Place the standards in the side slots next to the juice.

☐ 8. Cover the top of the block.

☐ 9. Allow light to enter the slots in the block by holding the block up to the light.

☐ 10. Choose the best color match.

☐ 11. Record the pH of the standard.

☐ 12. Continue this procedure until all substances are tested.

Lesson 26

Substance	pH
lemon juice	
boric acid	
vinegar	
HCl	
lye	
limewater	
baking soda	
$Mg(OH)_2$	

Questions for Review

1. Why is light necessary in this process?
2. What is a source of error in this procedure?

Laboratory Techniques

To learn how to use a pH Meter.

Background Information

An electrical machine is very sensitive to the H^+ and OH^- concentration of a solution. The machine has a very sensitive tube (electrode) which detects the presence of ions easily. This eliminates the errors which arise from the visual matching of colors. There is a scale or meter in the machine which allows you to read the pH directly in tenths.

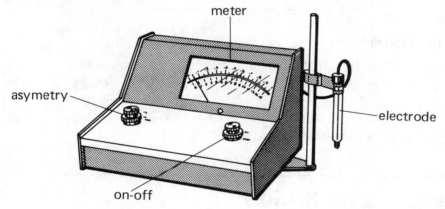

Procedure

I.   Meter Use.

☐   1. Switch the on-off switch to stand-by for several minutes before use.

☐   2. Place the electrode into a neutral buffer solution.

☐   3. Turn switch on to read.

☐   4. Read the result on the meter. Since the pH of the solution is 7, the needle of the meter should be on 7. If the needle is not on 7, turn the asymetry dial until the needle rests on 7. The machine is now calibrated. TURN TO STAND-BY.

☐   5. Wash the electrode in distilled water.

☐   6. Insert electrode into the solution to be tested.

☐   7. Turn dial to read.

☐   8. Read the meter.

☐ 9. Wash the electrode in distilled water when finished. The electrode must be washed after each use.

☐ 10. Continue the above procedure until all the substances have been tested. Record results on chart.

Substance	pH
lemon juice	
boric acid	
vinegar	
HC1	
lye	
limewater	
baking soda	
$Mg(OH)_2$	

II. Electrode Handling.

☐ 1. The electrode must be filled with a conducting fluid before use.

☐ 2. The opening on the side of the electrode is uncovered when the machine is in use.

☐ 3. Cover the opening with the rubber flap when not in use.

☐ 4. Store the electrode in water.

Questions for Review

1. Why is the electrode cleaned after each use?
2. Which method of pH determination is most accurate? Why?

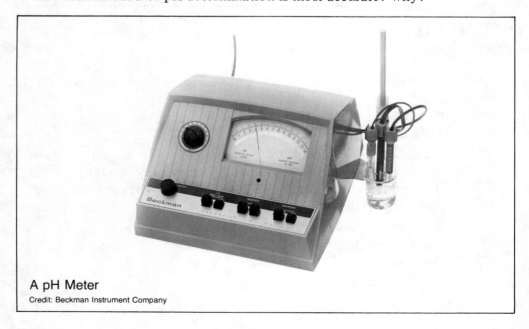

A pH Meter
Credit: Beckman Instrument Company

To learn how to read a thermometer.

Background Information

All living organisms live within a certain temperature range. They are either capable of maintaining a constant body temperature or they may keep themselves in an environment which does not lower or raise their body temperature appreciably. Certain bodily chemical reactions such as digestion require a specific temperature. A frog maintained at a low temperature becomes inactive as his body processes slow down. Because temperature is important to life, it is essential that you learn how to measure it.

A thermometer is the tool used to record temperature which is the measure of the amount of heat. The thermometer consists of a glass tube with a bulb at one end. Within the bulb is a liquid metal, mercury. All metals expand in heat and contract in the cold. The mercury will rise in the tube in the heat and descend in the cold.

In England and the U.S., temperature is recorded on a Fahrenheit (F°) scale. On this scale water boils at 212° and freezes at 32°. The more universally accepted Celsius (C°) or Centigrade scale is used in the laboratory. On this scale water boils at 100° and freezes at 0°. To convert from F to C a formula is used:

$$C = \frac{(F - 32°)}{1.8}$$

Procedure

☐ 1. Examine your thermometer. Locate the mercury in the glass tube. Hold a piece of cardboard behind the thermometer to make it easier to read the mercury. *Draw your thermometer.*

☐ 2. Suspend two thermometers in the classroom at heights of 2 ft. and 8 ft. *Read the temperature in both systems at the end of 5 minutes.*

☐ 3. Suspend a thermometer outside the window for 5 minutes. *Read the temperature in both systems.*

☐ 4. Place a thermometer in a pan of ice cubes. *Read and record temperature at the end of 5 minutes.*

☐ 5. Insert a thermometer into boiling water. *Read and record temperature at the end of 5 minutes.*

Lesson 28

Location	F°	C°
2 ft in class		
8 ft in class		
outside class		
ice		
boiling water		

Questions for Review

1. What is the maximum temperature which can be recorded by your thermometer in both systems?
2. What is body temperature in C° ?

To study the technique of paper chromatography.

Background Information

Chromatography is a process used to separate closely related substances in a solution. In this process a drop of the solution is placed on a piece of filter paper which touches a liquid such as alcohol or acetone. There is a special law which states that the liquid climbs or moves up the paper. This is the law of capillary action. As the liquid moves up the paper and through the solution, it takes some of the substances which were in the solution along with it. Not all the substances in the solution move with the same speed. The fast moving substances climb to the top of the paper faster than the slower moving ones. When the alcohol or acetone stop moving, the substances also stop moving. The different substances appear as bands or lines on different parts of the filter paper. In this way the substances are separated from one another.

A green leaf is green because it has a special pigment called chlorophyll in each cell. There are different types of chlorophylls as well as other colored pigments which cannot be seen because of the green color. To separate the different pigments, chromatography is used. In addition, there are many proteins in the body fluids which cannot be easily separated from each other. Chromatography allows for their separation. The type and abundance of proteins in the body fluids may be used as a diagnostic tool. Special machines have been designed along the lines of these principles for this reason.

Procedure

- ☐ 1. Cut a one inch wide strip of filter paper.
- ☐ 2. Place an eye hook into a rubber stopper. Place the filter paper on the hook.
- ☐ 3. Cut the end of the filter paper into a point.
- ☐ 4. Place spinach leaves and clean sand in a mortar along with 50 ml of acetone and grind until a green color appears.
- ☐ 5. Filter the material.
- ☐ 6. Pour 9 ml of petroleum ether into a test tube.
- ☐ 7. Add 1 ml of acetone to the test tube.
- ☐ 8. Place one drop of the filtered material with a micro-pipette or tooth pick a few millimeters from the pointed end of the filter paper.
- ☐ 9. Let the drop dry.
- ☐ 10. Place a second drop of the filtered material on the same spot as the first drop.

☐ 11. Let dry.

☐ 12. Place a third drop on the same spot as the second.

☐ 13. Let dry.

☐ 14. Place the pointed end of the filter paper into the test tube of ether and acetone. Only the tip should touch the liquid.

☐ 15. In about 10 minutes bands of orange and green should appear. The separation is completed.

☐ 16. Follow the same procedure but this time spot the filter paper with ink from a Bic pen (red or blue ink).

Questions for Review

1. Why is chromatography a useful tool?
2. How could you use chromatography to separate proteins?

The Compound Microscope

The microscope is an extension of man's eyes because it allows him to see things which are too small to be seen with the naked eye.

If you look carefully at your microscope, you will notice the eyepiece (OCULAR). The eyepiece contains an enlarging lens. At the base of a rotating piece (NOSE PIECE) there are two OBJECTIVES. In each objective there is another series of magnifying lenses. Since you can only use one objective at a time along with the ocular, you are using two lenses to enlarge a specimen. The word compound means the use of two lenses.

Notice the numbers etched into the ocular and objectives. The magnification is determined by multiplying the number on the ocular by the number on the objective. Notice the difference in the size of the objectives. The greater the magnification of the objective, the longer it is.

The large knob is used to focus under Low Power (COARSE ADJUSTMENT). Low Power (LP) refers to the 100X magnification of your microscope. To obtain this magnification, the 10X objective is used. The small know (FINE ADJUSTMENT) is used exclusively under High Power (HP) and sometimes under low power.

A small wheel on the left side of the stage (DIAPHRAGM) controls the size of the opening in the stage. The STAGE is the part of the microscope where the slide is placed. Turn the wheel and observe what happens.

You will also notice a MIRROR with two surfaces just above the BASE and below the diaphragm. Look into the ocular after the low power objective has been rotated over the stage. Move the mirror while you are looking into the microscope. What do you notice?

The portion of the microscope which connects the ocular to the objectives is known as the BARREL. That part which connects the barrel and the focusing mechanism to the stage is known as the ARM.

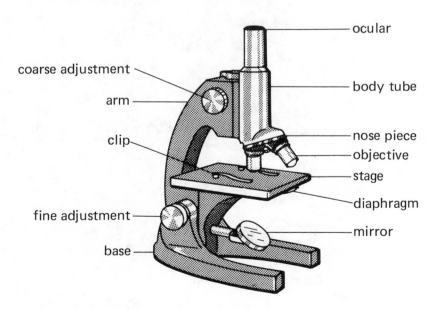

Complete this chart.

Part	Function of the part
ocular	
barrel	
nose piece	
LP objective	
HP objective	
stage	
clips	
coarse adjustment	
fine adjustment	
arm	
mirror	
diaphragm	
base	

Locate and label each part of the microscope.

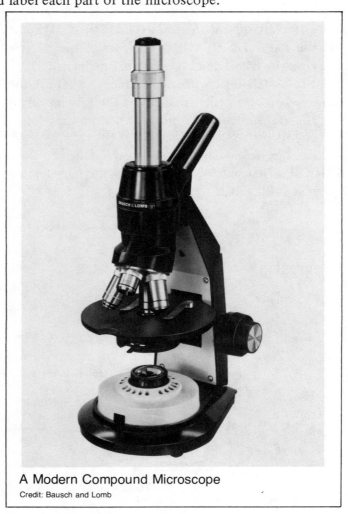

A Modern Compound Microscope
Credit: Bausch and Lomb

To study how to use the microscope.

Procedure

- ☐ 1. Do not touch the eyepiece with your eyelashes.
- ☐ 2. Keep both eyes open while using the microscope.

I. Focusing - LP.

- ☐ 1. Turn the LP objective until it clicks into place over the hole in the stage.
- ☐ 2. Open the diaphragm so that the number 5 is visible (maximum opening).
- ☐ 3. Turn the mirror so that the flat side faces the stage.
- ☐ 4. With your eye at the ocular move the mirror until the best possible light is obtained. White light not blue or pink is needed.
- ☐ 5. Place a slide on the stage. The object should be in the center.
- ☐ 6. With your eyes at the level of the stage, turn the coarse adjustment knob until the objective is 1/4 of an inch above the slide.
- ☐ 7. Place your eye at the ocular. Raise the objective by turning the coarse adjustment towards you. Never focus down on a slide.
- ☐ 8. If you cannot locate the object, repeat step 6 and 7.
- ☐ 9. Once you have the object in focus, you may use the fine adjustment knob to make the picture sharper. Turn the knob *very* slowly.

II. Focusing - HP.

- ☐ 1. Focus under LP first.
- ☐ 2. Turn the nosepiece so that the high power objective clicks into place. Do *not* touch the coarse adjustment knob.
- ☐ 3. With your eye at the eyepiece, turn the *fine adjustment* very slowly until the image is cleared.
- ☐ 4. If you have trouble finding the object, start all over again by following all the steps in LP focusing first then switch to HP.

IMPORTANT THINGS TO REMEMBER

- ☐ 1. You must always find the object under LP before examining the slide under HP.
- ☐ 2. You must always be sure to see that you have the best possible light before examining the slide.
- ☐ 3. *Never* focus with the coarse adjustment under HP. *Use fine adjustment only*.

Lesson 30

☐   4.   You can use fine adjustment with any power on your microscope.

☐   5.   Clean the lenses and mirror *before* and *after* use with lens paper.

III. Depth of Objects.

☐   1.   Very gently turn your fine adjustment knob. Observe that the barrel moves.

☐   2.   Notice that on the right side of the microscope near the fine adjustment knob, there is a small scale of lines.

☐   3.   Focus on the top of the object. Observe the position of the lines.

☐   4.   Focus on the bottom of the object. Observe the position of the lines.

☐   5.   The distance between each line is usually indicated on the barrel. The distance you moved the fine adjustment knob gives you the thickness of the specimen.

☐   6.   Multiply that answer by 1000 to convert mm to microns.

Questions for Review

1. Why must you keep your eyelashes off the eyepiece?
2. Why do you focus with the fine adjustment knob under HP?
3. Why must the lenses be clean?
4. Why must you always have the best possible light?

Background Information

Before you begin to examine slides, there are a few important facts to learn about the microscope.

Procedure

☐ 1. Place the letter "a" slide on the stage in such a way that the letter is facing you exactly as you would read it.

☐ 2. Draw the letter as you see it under low power.

☐ 3. Move the slide towards you. What happens to the image?

☐ 4. Move the slide away from you. What happens to the image?

☐ 5. Move the slide to the right and then to the left. What happens to the image?

☐ 6. Turn to high power. What happened to the light? Why?

☐ 7. Draw the letter "a" as seen under high power.

Questions for Review

1. What differences do you notice in the appearance of the letter "a" under low and high power?
2. In what 3 ways is the letter "a" seen with the microscope different from the letter seen with the naked eye?
3. Do you see more of the letter under low or high power?
4. Is the letter largest under low or high power?
5. Examine the diameter of the objectives. What is the relationship between the size of the diameter and the magnification?
6. Why would you see less under high power?
7. Why does the slide appear darker under high power?

Problem
To study some plant cells.

Background Information

Most microscopic work involves the preparation of slides. A specimen must be placed on a slide in such a way that you are able to see as much detail as possible. This means that the specimen must be very thin. In many instances, a stain must be used to reveal much of the detailed structure. After the slides are properly prepared, observation is possible.

Procedure

☐1. With tweezers, remove a very thin piece of tissue from the inside of a piece of celery.
☐2. Place a small piece of this membrane on a glass slide. Add a drop of water and cover with a cover slip.
☐3. Observe under LP. The box-like structures are cells. The granular portion is the cytoplasm and the dark, round body is the nucleus.
☐4. Make a drawing of several cells.
☐5. Observe under HP. *Determine the thickness of the cells. Make a drawing of several cells.*

Staining

☐1. Place a drop of iodine against one side of the cover slip.
☐2. Place a piece of lens paper against the opposite side of the cover slip. The lens paper will draw the water towards it while the iodine will also be drawn across the slide.
☐3. Observe under LP and draw a few cells.
☐4. Observe under HP and draw a few cells. What changes do you notice in the appearance of the cells?

Spinach and Lettuce Slides

☐1. Prepare slides of spinach and lettuce cells.
☐2. Follow the exact procedures as above. Use different stains.

Laboratory Techniques

Questions for Review

1. What change did you notice between the stained and unstained slides?
2. What do the stains do?
3. Why must the specimens on the slide be very thin?

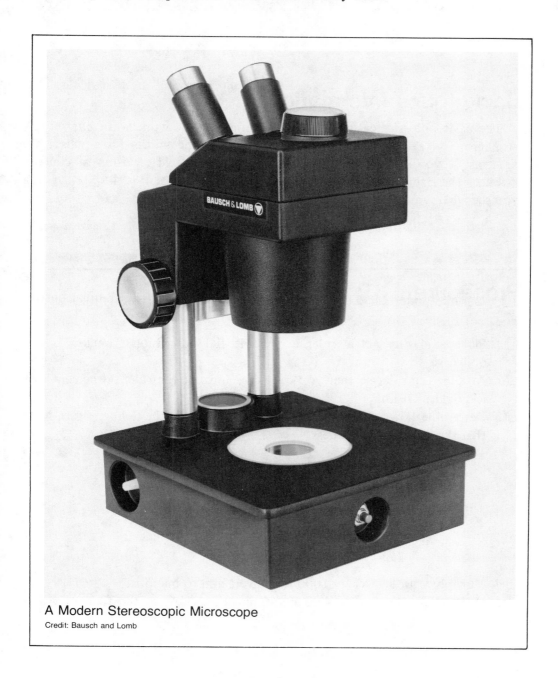

A Modern Stereoscopic Microscope
Credit: Bausch and Lomb

To learn how to measure length and width of the specimen under a microscope.

Problem

Lesson 33

Background Information

The basic unit of measurement used in microscopic work is the *micron* (u). A micron is 1/1000 of a millimeter. Therefore, one millimeter equals 1000 microns. If you know how many microns wide the field of vision is, you can estimate the size of observed specimens. The *field of vision* is the circular area you see when you look through the ocular.

Procedure

Width of Field of Vision

☐ 1. Place a plastic metric ruler across the field of vision. Use low power objective.

☐ 2. Arrange the ruler so that you can see 2 lines of the ruler in the center of the field of vision.

☐ 3. Determine how much more than 1 mm (two lines) the field really is. Note that the lines have thickness.

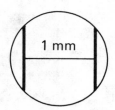

☐ 4. Multiply your answer by 1000 to convert mm to microns.

☐ 5. Divide your answer by 4 to determine the width of the field of vision under high power.

Use of Information

☐ 1. Place a slide on the stage. Find out (estimate) how many specimens placed end to end would stretch across the field.

☐ 2. Divide this number into 1500u under LP.

☐ 3. Under HP follow the same procedure but divide the number of specimens into 375u.

Example:

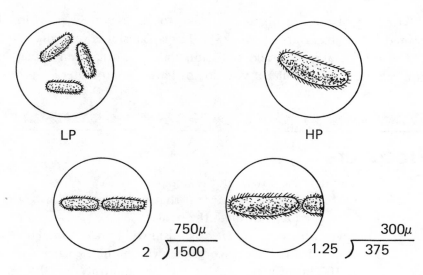

LP   HP

$$2\ \overline{)\ 1500}^{\ 750\mu}$$ $$1.25\ \overline{)\ 375}^{\ 300\mu}$$

Question for Review

1. Why is the length and width of organisms important to know?

Problem	# To learn how to determine length and width by using a metric ruler.

Background Information

With very large organisms it is easy to use the field of vision method to estimate their size. But with very small organisms, it is very difficult to estimate how many fit across a field of vision unless you have an ocular micrometer. You can use a metric ruler if you do not have a micrometer.

Procedure

☐ 1. Focus under low power on the organism.
☐ 2. Place a ruler across the stage so that you can see it with one eye while the other eye looks through the ocular.
☐ 3. Your eyes will cross and the organism will appear to fall on the ruler.
☐ 4. Count how many lines the organism covers on the ruler.
☐ 5. Divide 100 into the number of lines and multiply by 1000.

OR

Multiply the number of lines by 10.
☐ 6. To find the width, turn the ruler in a verticle position and follow the same rules.
☐ 7. Click the high power objective into place and focus.
☐ 8. Place the ruler across the stage so that you can see it.
☐ 9. Count the number of lines that the organism covers on the ruler.
☐10. Divide 400 into the number of lines and multiply by 1000.

OR

Multiply the number of lines by 2.5.

Questions for Review

1. Which method of measuring size is the easier? Why?
2. Which method is better? Why?
3. Why do you divide by 100 and multiply by 1000 under LP to get the right size?
4. Why do you divide by 400 and multiply by 1000 under HP to get an answer?

To learn how to calibrate an ocular micrometer.

Background Information

To accurately measure an object under a microscope, a special eyepiece with a scale drawn on it is used. An *ocular micrometer* is a small glass disc with a small scale ruled into it.

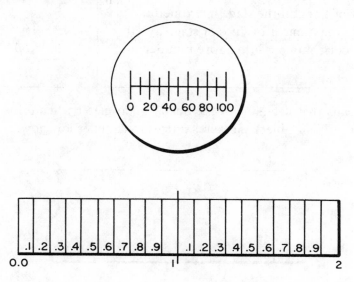

Look into your microscope and examine the ocular micrometer. Switch from low to high power. Notice that this has no effect on the ocular micrometer. Under low power an object may measure 20 units or fill the field from 0 to 20 on the scale. Under high power the same object is enlarged more so that it may only fill 10 units (0 to 10) on the scale. We would then get two different measurements for the same object. In order to get an accurate measurement, you must find out how large one unit on the scale is for low power and high power (calibration). To do this you need to use a stage micrometer. The stage micrometer is a ruled slide in which the value of each line is known.

Lesson 35

Procedure

☐ 1. Draw the ocular micrometer.
☐ 2. Draw the stage micrometer.
☐ 3. Place the stage micrometer on the stage of the microscope and focus under low power.
☐ 4. Line up the 0.0 line of the stage micrometer with the 0 line of the ocular micrometer.
☐ 5. Look to see where there is a match between the two scales.
☐ 6. Complete this chart (number refers to the matching points).

number of lines on the ocular micrometer	5
number of lines on the stage micrometer	3
multiply the number of lines of stage by 10	$3 \times 10 = 30\mu$
divide ocular number into above number	$\dfrac{30}{5} = 6\mu$

7. This means that each line of the ocular micrometer when using low power equals 6u. If an object measures 2 lines long under low power, it is 2 x 6u = 12u.

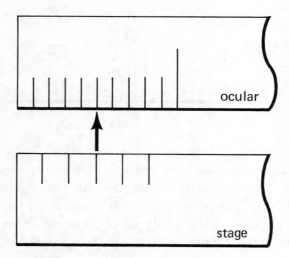

To learn to calibrate the ocular micrometer under HP.

Background Information

The calibration of the ocular micrometer under HP follows the same procedure as under LP. However, the value for each line of the micrometer will be different.

Procedure

☐1. Focus under low power first.
☐2. Click the high power objective into place.
☐3. Match the 0.0 line of the stage micrometer to the 0 line of the ocular micrometer. *CAUTION: Focus with fine adjustment only.*
☐4. Find a match between the two scales.
☐5. Complete this chart.

number of lines on ocular micrometer	20
number of lines on the stage micrometer	3
multiply line of stage x 10	30
divide ocular number into above number	$\dfrac{30}{20} = 1.5\mu$

☐6. This means that each line under high power is equal to 1.5. If an object measure 2 lines under high power, it is 3 lines long.

Lesson 36

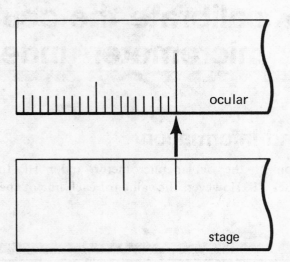

ocular

stage

Questions for Review

1. Which method discussed so far is the most accurate means of measuring length and width?
2. Why is the size of an organism important to know?

To practice the techniques of microscopic measurement.

Background Information

In order to practice the techniques of microscopic measurement, you will be given some prepared slides. In addition you will prepare some slides yourself.

Procedure

☐ 1. Place a few grains of salt in the center of a clean slide. Measure under low and high power with all three methods.

☐ 2. Remove a piece of human hair and place in the center of a clean slide. Cover with a cover slip. Measure the length and width under low and high power.

☐ 3. Examine a prepared blood cell slide. Measure the length and width of each type of cell.

☐ 4. There are several slides of different kinds of threads. Notice that the threads have been criss-crossed so that geometric boxes are formed on the slide. Measure the length and width of each box as well as the thickness of each kind of thread. Make sure that you record the letter of your slide, so that you can check your answer against the teacher's answer key.

☐ 5. Complete this chart.

Object	Method of Measurement	Size (HP)
salt		
hair		
blood cells		
threads		

Questions for Review

1. Which method of measurement is the easiest?
2. Which method of measurement is the most accurate?
3. Why are the results of measurements different in each method?

Problem To learn how to use an oil immersion lens.

Background Information

When examining certain slides such as bacteria, note that the organisms are so small that they are difficult to see even under high power. It is very difficult to distinguish any of their details. In order to enlarge the organisms a special lens, oil immersion, is used.

This lens is immersed in oil. The oil bends the rays of light into the objective. This is necessary because the objective opening is very small. Since the objective opening is so small, not enough light can pass through. The oil serves to direct the light into the small opening. The oil immersion lens will magnify objects at least 970 X.

Procedure

☐ 1. Place a microscope lamp under the stage of a microscope with an oil immersion lens. Plug in.

☐ 2. Obtain the maximum amount of light. Control with the diaphragm or condenser.

☐ 3. Place the slide on the stage.

☐ 4. Focus on the area you wish to see under low power and then high power.

☐ 5. Raise the objectives so that they are at least 3/4 of an inch off the stage.

☐ 6. Place one drop of oil on the slide.

☐ 7. Rotate the oil immersion lens into place.

☐ 8. With your eye at the stage, bring the oil immersion lens down into the drop of oil.

☐ 9. When you see a flash of light, you know that the oil immersion lens has made contact with the oil. *Do not ram the lens into the slide.*

☐10. Focus with *fine adjustment* only.

☐11. When you are finished using the lens, clean with a little xylol applied to a piece of lens paper.

☐12. Examine blood and bacterial slides (commercially prepared).

Questions for Review

1. What is the power of your oil immersion lens?
2. How do you know the power of the lens?
3. Why do we use lamps?
4. What is the advantage of using oil immersion?

Lesson 38

TEST YOURSELF

1. What is the pH of water?
2. In what pH range is an acid found?
3. What color does litmus paper turn in a base?
4. What is body temperature in $C°$?
5. By what process are closely related substances separated from each other?
6. If an organism under LP covers 6 lines on the ocular micrometer, how large is it?
7. What is the basic unit of microscopic measurement?
8. If an organism under HP covers 2 lines on the ocular micrometer, how large is it?
9. What type of lens must be used to enlarge a specimen 1000X?
10. What are some common stains used in preparing slides for microscopic study?

1. _____
2. _____
3. _____
4. _____
5. _____
6. _____
7. _____
8. _____
9. _____
10. _____

Answers

1. 7
2. 7 to 1
3. red to blue
4. $37°$
5. chromatography
6. 36u
7. micron
8. 3u
9. oil immersion
10. methylene blue iodine

Glossary

analytical balance   A special scale with 0.0001g accuracy.

bunsen burner   A burner which produces a high temperature without soot.

centimeter   A measure of length.

chromatography   A technique used to separate closely related substances from each other.

compound microscope   A light microscope.

dial-o-gram   Special scale with .01g accuracy.

electrode   A tube that detects small electrical charges.

flanging   Process of strengthening the edges of glassware.

fire polishing   A process of smoothing the edges of rough glassware.

graduate glassware   Glassware in which known gradations are etched into its side.

indicator   A substance that detects the presence of hydrogen ions.

liter   A measure of volume.

meter   A measure of length.

metric system   A system used in scientific measurements.

micron   A measure of length .001 of a mm.

micrometer-ocular   Ruled scale in the ocular of a microscope.

micrometer-stage   A ruled scale on a slide used on the stage of a microscope.

milliliter   A measure of volume, 1/1000 of a liter.

millimeter   A measure of length, 1/1000 of a meter.

oil immersion   A microscopic lens that can be immersed in oil.

percentage solution   A solution whose concentration is measured per 100 cc.

pH   A measure of the hydrogen ion concentration of a solution.

pH meter   An electrical device for the measure of the hydrogen ion concentration in a solution.

pipette   A graduate glass tube used to transfer or measure specific amounts of liquids.

solute   Particles which are to be dissolved in a solution.

solution   A mixture of solute in a solvent.

solvent   A dissolving agent for a solute.

stain   A dye which is used to color materials on a slide.

thermometer   A device for the measurement of temperature.

triple beam balance   A scale which weights to the .1g

volume   The capacity of a container.

Unit II

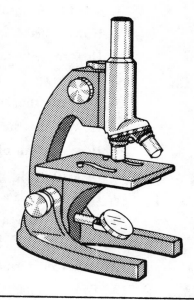

Hematology

Unit II Table of Contents

To the Student

We live in an exciting time. Men have walked on the moon. Others have been given a second chance for life with transplanted organs. Today, many of the diseases which plagued man no longer affect us. How many of you have heard of polio? Twenty years ago, it was one of the major causes of death in young children. In spite of man's progress towards the conquest of disease, it is still with us. However, one of the reasons for man's increased life span is the speedy diagnosis and treatment of disease.

Who performs the diagnostic tests, interprets their results, and prescribes a treatment? You can be one of these key people who strive to keep man healthy! This book has been written to introduce you to some of the many diagnostic tools used to determine the state of man's health. There are many aspects of diagnostic tests. This unit deals with hematology. At the completion of this unit, you will have some ideas of how the simple blood tests are performed and what is the significance of their results. Even if you do not pursue a medical career, this unit will give you a better understanding of the functioning of your complex human body.

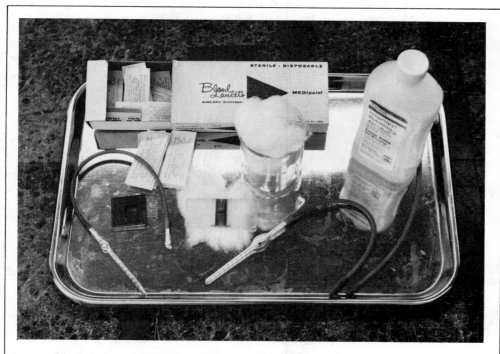

A Laboratory Set Up For Blood Cell Counting

Hematology

PATH OF THE BLOOD

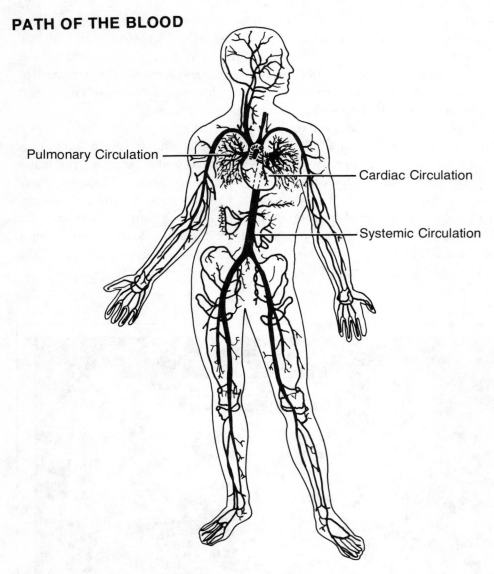

Pulmonary Circulation

Cardiac Circulation

Systemic Circulation

Preface

Blood is the life fluid of the body. It has many functions. It carries oxygen to the cells and gaseous wastes, carbon dioxide, away. It carries nutritive materials to all the cells and metabolic wastes to the kidneys. It protects the body against invading organisms and helps to maintain body temperature.

Blood consists of a fluid, *plasma,* in which cells are suspended. Ninety percent of the plasma is water. In addition, plasma is composed of various proteins, antibodies, nutritive materials (amino acids, carbohydrates), and salts. The cellular elements consist of red and white blood cells and platelets.

Laboratory Techniques

Hematology is the study of the blood. It deals primarily with the cellular elements, their number, their types, and the presence of abnormal cells or features. A change in any of the normal elements may be due to disease or organic disorders. Analysis of the blood enables one to determine and confirm abnormal bodily conditions.

Blood Cells

There are various types of blood cells. The most numerous and the smallest are red blood cells. As the name implies, these cells are red in color. The color is due to the presence of hemoglobin. Hemoglobin is a complex protein combined with a metallic element, iron. Its structure is similar to the chlorophyll molecule.

The hemoglobin is responsible for carrying oxygen to the cells of the body. A lack of hemoglobin, a distortion in the red blood cell, or the decrease in the number of red blood cells impairs the oxygen carrying capacity.

There are several types of white blood cells, *leukocytes*. In general, these cells protect the body from foreign protein or organisms.

Neutrophils and monocytes demonstrate *amoeboid* properties. They move and engulf materials like the ameba. There are usually more neutrophils in the blood than monocytes. The monocytes move very slowly through the body tissues but have a great *phagocytic* (engulfing) capacity while the neutrophils move rapidly but do not engulf as many foreign particles per cell.

Eosinophils may act to detoxify foreign proteins. This means that they neutralize and render these proteins harmless.

Basophils may produce heparin. Heparin is a substance which prevents the blood from clotting in the blood vessels. Interestingly, heparin is found in snake venom.

It has been suggested that lymphocytes may be able to produce antibodies or antitoxins which neutralize bacterial organisms or their poisons.

Platelets, on the other hand, are involved in the complex blood clotting mechanism. Because of their presence a clot will form when the blood vessels are cut or damaged. They help to prevent a person from bleeding to death.

The story of the development of blood cells, hematopoiesis, is extremely complex and not fully understood. Several areas of the body give rise to the cells that eventually mature into blood cells. In adults these areas include the bone tissues of the sternum (breast bone), pelvic area (hips), vertebrae (back bone), skull, ribs, clavicles (shoulders), and the long bones (legs and arms).

It is through the examination of these blood cells that disease or organic disorders may be detected and treated.

Problem   To study a blood smear (prepared slide).

Background Information

Since there are different types of blood cells, a brief description of each follows so that you may identify them easily.

The RED BLOOD CELL or ERYTHROCYTE appears buff-pink on the edges while the center has little stain.

There are several different kinds of WHITE BLOOD CELLS, WBC. An EOSINOPHIL is very round and appears very granular. The granules stain bright reddish-orange. The nucleus appears to have two lobes.

A NEUTROPHIL is about two times as large as a RBC. The cytoplasm appears pinkish and the nucleus is composed of several lobes connected by very thin bands.

A LYMPHOCYTE stains blue and the nucleus appears as a large dark mass.

A MONOCYTE stains blue and the nucleus appears as a dark mass with a slight indentation.

A BASOPHIL appears as a cluster of small round dark bodies.

Procedure

☐ 1. Follow the rules for oil immersion and examine the slide.
☐ 2. Draw the different types of cells.
☐ 3. Measure the size of the different types of cells with any method you learned.
☐ 4. Complete the chart.

Blood Cell	Size

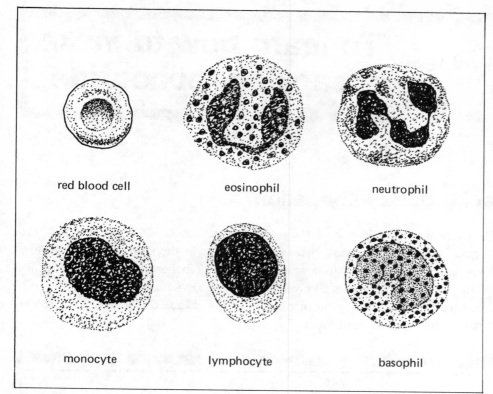

red blood cell   eosinophil   neutrophil

monocyte   lymphocyte   basophil

Fig. 1

Questions for Review

1. Why is oil immersion used?
2. What did the stain do to the blood cells?
3. Which blood cells are most numerous?
4. Which blood cells are the largest?
5. What unit of measurement is used?

Lesson 2

Problem
To learn how to make a capillary puncture.

Background Information

Capillary puncture is one of the most common methods of collecting blood. It is easy, simple, causes very little pain and fear in the patient. It can be done quickly and does not require as much skill as other methods. The blood collected in this way is less likely to be distorted. Several places of the body can be used for a capillary puncture such as the ear lobe or the tip of the finger. The tip of the finger is used most frequently.

Procedure

☐ 1. Wash your hands before you begin.
☐ 2. The finger tip should be warm.
☐ 3. Rub the finger tip with cotton soaked in alcohol to remove dirt and germs.
☐ 4. Hold the finger in one hand and apply gentle pressure to hold the skin tight.
☐ 5. Hold the sterile hemalet in the other hand.
☐ 6. A finger puncture should be made along the side of the finger tip. More nerve endings are found on the finger print area of the finger, therefore, more pain results.
☐ 7. The puncture should be made with a quick, firm jab, 3-4 mm in depth.
☐ 8. The first drop of blood that appears is wiped away.
☐ 9. The blood should not be squeezed out because it will mix with the tissue fluid.
☐10. The second drop will be pipetted or allowed to fall on to a slide.

Questions for Review

1. What will happen if the finger is not cleaned with alcohol?
2. Why do we not use the first drop of blood?
3. Why is the capillary puncture most frequently used?

Problem To study how to make a blood smear.

Lesson **3**

Background Information

In order to examine blood cells, it is necessary to collect and prepare a drop of blood for examination.

Procedure

☐ 1. Make a finger puncture – FOLLOW ALL RULES FOR FINGER PUNCTURE.

☐ 2. Place a slide on a flat surface. Clean slide with alcohol.

☐ 3. Place a drop of blood on the clean glass slide about 3/4 of an inch from one end.

☐ 4. Place a second slide with one end at a 30° angle on the first slide. Hold the slide with the thumb and index finger.

☐ 5. Draw the second slide (spreader) towards the drop of blood until contact is made.

☐ 6. Allow the blood to spread evenly under the narrow edge of the spreader.

☐ 7. With a fast but smooth gliding movement, push the spreader over the slide in the opposite direction. (picture on right)

☐ 8. Let the slide dry in the air (air dry). Do *not* blow on it.

☐ 9. Practice this procedure with a molasses solution before you make a finger puncture.

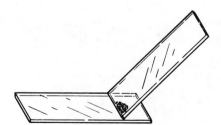 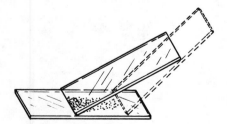

Lesson 3

Questions for Review

1. Why is the slide called a smear?
2. Why is the slide cleaned with alcohol?
3. Why must a continuous, quick stroke be used in preparing the smear?

Problem
To study how to stain a blood smear.

Background Information

In order to see the blood cells and to distinguish the different types, a stain is necessary. Wright's stain is the stain used to color the blood cells of the smear.

Procedure

- ☐ 1. Place the slide on a staining tray.
- ☐ 2. Add 25 to 40 drops of Wright's stain. This should cover the whole slide.
- ☐ 3. Let the slide stand for 1 to 3 minutes.
- ☐ 4. Add about 20 drops of buffer solution (distilled water) so that it is evenly spread on the whole slide.
- ☐ 5. Mix the two solutions on the slide by gently blowing on several sides. A silvery scum will float to the top of the slide.
- ☐ 6. Allow to set for 4 minutes. A greenish metallic scum should appear. The edges show a reddish tint.
- ☐ 7. Wash off the excess staining solution by allowing cold water to run over the slide gently. The slide must remain in a flat position. The washing takes 5 to 30 seconds until the thinner portion of the film becomes yellow or pink.
- ☐ 8. Wipe off the back of the slide.
- ☐ 9. The excess water is drained by tilting the slide and touching a blotter to the lower edge.
- ☐ 10. Allow the slide to air dry in a tilted position.

Questions for Review

1. Why must stains be used?
2. Why is the length of time a stain is allowed to stand important?

To study the structure Problem of a counting chamber (hemacytometer).

Lesson 5

Background Information

Normal blood contains a certain number of RBC and WBC. Usually there are 5 million RBC and 6000 WBC per drop of blood. An abnormal number, too much or too little, indicates a diseased condition. In order to determine the number of blood cells, a blood count must be taken. A hemacytometer is a chamber which makes the counting of blood cells possible. You must become familiar with the hemacytometer before you can properly use it.

Procedure

☐1. You will notice that there are two sides to the hemacytometer, one side is depressed and the other is a single piece of glass with an H shaped pattern.

☐2. Hold the hemacytometer up to the light and notice the lines etched in the glass. There are two areas which contain the etching. These areas are found between the boundaries of the H.

☐3. Place the hemacytometer on the stage of a microscope, depression side down on the stage.

☐4. Place a cover slip over the chamber.

☐5. Very carefully lower the *LOW POWER* objective until it touches the hemacytometer. *Keep your eye at the level of the stage.* Be careful not to crack the cover slip or the hemacytometer.

☐6. Looking through the ocular move the hemacytometer until the lines appear. You will have to move the body tube up to focus on the lines. There is a relatively high focus. *Never focus down on the hemacytometer.*

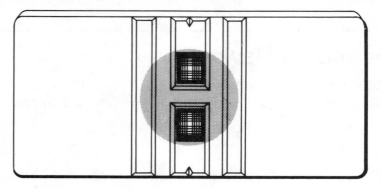

☐ 7. Focus with the fine adjustment when the lines are in view.

☐ 8. Carefully switch to **HIGH POWER**. Focus only with the *FINE ADJUSTMENT*.

☐ 9. Make sure that you can locate each major and minor square shown on this page.

Lesson 5

There are 9 major divisions each 1 mm square. Each major division is sub-divided. Notice that there is a central area in the shape of a cross where the divisions are very small.

In the very center there are 25 smaller areas. Each of these divisions is further subdivided into 16 squares. There are 400 squares in the central area. Each of the 400 squares is .0025 mm.

Questions for Review

1. Why are there large and small divisions?
2. What does the size of the squares tell us about the size of the blood cells?

To learn how to use the Thoma pipette.

Background Information

To dilute blood and other fluids the Thoma type of pipette is used. This pipette has a graduated capillary tube with a mark at the 0.5 and 1 unit, and a mixing bulb above the capillary tube. There is a red bead in the mixing bulb. Above the red bead is a shorter capillary tube marked 101. This pipette is used for red blood cell counts. Another pipette with a white bead and a capillary tube above the mixing bulb marked 11 is used for white blood cell counts. Because the blood is so thick, the cells stick together. The blood must be mixed with a fluid to separate the cells so that they can be counted. The Thoma pipette allows you to mix the blood with a fluid.

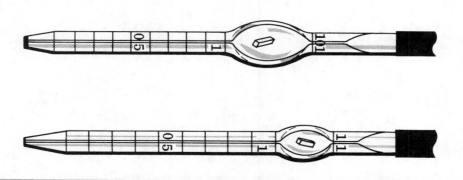

Procedure

☐ 1. Place the rubber tube on the end of the pipette so that it covers the area above the 101 mark or the 11 mark.
☐ 2. Place the tip of the pipette on the surface of a beaker holding a solution of molasses.
☐ 3. Hold the pipette in one hand between the thumb and index finger.
☐ 4. Place the plastic mouth piece in your mouth.
☐ 5. Draw the solution up to the 0.5 mark.
☐ 6. Wipe the tip with cotton.
☐ 7. Continue to practice this until you are able to reach the 0.5 mark.
☐ 8. After reaching the 0.5 mark, place the tip of the pipette into a beaker of water and draw the water to the 101 or 11 mark.
☐ 9. Practice until you are able to carry out this operation without trapping air bubbles in the pipette.

☐ 10. To discharge the pipette one drop at a time, place your finger over the opposite end of the pipette.

☐ 11. Remove the rubber tube and place your pointing finger over the opening. This will allow you to hold the pipette between the index and the thumb.

☐ 12. Practice discharging the solution a drop at a time.

Questions for Review

1. Why is such a small pipette used for drawing blood?
2. Why must you have exact control over the material in the pipette?

Problem To learn how to clean blood counting equipment.

Background Information

Pipettes and hemacytometers must be cleaned after use or the blood will clot making them impossible to reuse.

Procedure

Pipette cleaning

☐ 1. Draw water through the pipette by using a suction apparatus.
☐ 2. Insert the pipette into a hole on the rubber disc.
☐ 3. Insert the aspirator over a faucet and attach to the disc.
☐ 4. Place the rubber disc over a plastic container filled with water.
☐ 5. Turn water on for a few minutes. If clots remain in the pipette, remove with specially purchased fine wire.

Hemacytometer

☐ 1. Wash counting chamber and cover slip with water immediately after use.
☐ 2. Dry with soft cloth.

Question for Review

1. Why is just plain soap and water not used in cleaning the pipettes or hemacytometer?

Lesson 8

Background Information

The normal number of WBC varies from 5000 to 10,000 per cubic milliliter (drop) of blood. The number varies according to the time of day, nutritional conditions, and disease. If there is a permanent increase, this is called leukemia.

Bacteria and poisons are capable of attracting large numbers of WBC. This temporary increase in numbers may indicate the presence of infection.

Procedure

☐ 1. Make a finger puncture.
☐ 2. Draw blood through the white bead Thoma pipette up to the .5 mark.
☐ 3. Wipe off the excess blood from the pipette with a piece of cotton.
☐ 4. Draw a 2% acetic acid solution to the 11 mark. This destroys the RBC.
☐ 5. Hold the pipette upright to prevent air bubbles. Mix the contents by rotating the pipette gently.
☐ 6. Fill the hemacytometer

    a. Remove the mouth piece and place your finger over the opening.
    b. Mix the material for 2 minutes by shaking the pipette in a figure eight motion. Hold the pipette between the thumb and index finger.
    c. Place a cover slip over the hemacytometer. Discard 5 drops of blood from the pipette.
    d. Hold the pipette at a 45° angle and touch the pipette to the place where the cover slip meets the counting chamber.
    e. Allow the material to flow under the cover slip into the counting chamber. No fluid should overflow out of the chamber.
    f. Fill the counting chamber on the other side.
    g. Allow to settle for 2-3 minutes.
    h. Focus under Low Power then switch to High Power.

☐ 7. Count

    a. Use the upper and lower corners of the counting chamber, the parts labelled 1, 3, 5, and 7.
    b. Count the cells in each of the squares following a counting pattern.

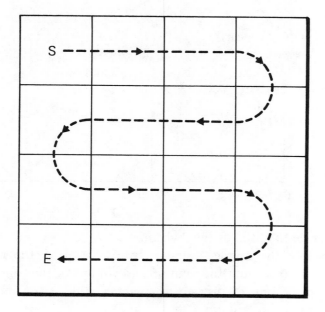

c. Count the cells lying within each square and those touching the upper and right hand lines of each square. Do not count those touching the left hand and lower lines. Example—there are 12 cells in this section of the hemacytometer.

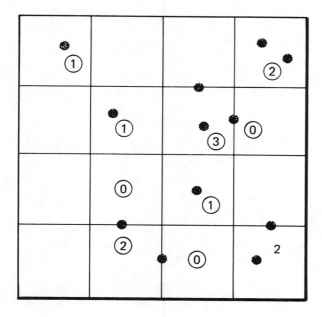

Lesson 8

d. Complete this chart.

Chamber I	No. of cells	Chamber II	No. of cells
square 1 square 3 square 5 square 7			

total

e. Average the total of the 2 chambers.

f. Multiply the average number by 50. 50 is the number which takes into account the dilution and volume of the counting chamber.

☐ 8. You may find it useful to practice the entire procedure with a yeast-molasses solution.

Questions for Review

1. Why do you discard the first few drops of blood?
2. Why are the larger squares used for counting WBC?

How to take a red blood cell count.

Background Information

A healthy male has 5 million RBC/cu. ml of blood (drop), and a female has 4½ million RBC. A decrease in red blood cells may indicate a disease such as anemia.

Procedure

☐ 1. Make a finger puncture.

☐ 2. Draw blood to the .5 mark through the red bead Thoma pipette.

☐ 3. Wipe off the excess blood from the pipette with a piece of cotton.

☐ 4. Draw a diluting fluid to the 101 mark. A diluting fluid not only thins out the blood but also destroys the white blood cells and platelets. Hayems or Toisons fluid is most often used.

☐ 5. Hold the pipette in a vertical position and turn slightly to avoid the forming of air bubbles. Mix the contents by rotating the pipette gently.

☐ 6. Fill the hemacytometer — follow the procedures used in making white blood cell count.

☐ 7. Count

a. Find the central area of the hemacytometer — the one with the 400 small squares. Count all the RBC located in the 5 squares marked a. b. c. d. and e.

b. Follow the same counting procedures as for the white blood cells.

c. Complete this chart.

Chamber I	No. of cells	Chamber II	No. of cells
square a square b square c square d square e			

total

d. Average the total of both chambers. _____

e. Multiply the average number 200 x 10 x 5 _____

or

Just add four zeros to the average number _____

Questions for Review

1. Why is a diluting fluid used?
2. Why must you avoid the formation of air bubbles?
3. Why are the two sides of the hemacytometer used?
4. Why are the first few drops of blood discarded?

How to make a differerential WBC count .

Background Information

In certain disease conditions there is an increase or decrease in the different types of WBC. In addition to knowing the entire number of WBC, it is important to know the percent of the different kinds that are present. The ascertaining of the percent of the types of WBC is known as a *differential count*.

Procedure

☐ 1. Prepare a blood smear.
☐ 2. Stain the smear following the Wright stain procedure.
☐ 3. Count 100 consecutive WBC.
☐ 4. Tabulate the type as you count.
☐ 5. Complete this chart.

Type of WBC	number counted	percent
lymphocyte		
monocyte		
neutrophil		
eosinophil		
basophil		

total

6. Determine the percent of each type.

Question for Review

1. How does the result obtained from the class compare to the average expected result?

Lesson 10

TEST YOURSELF

1. What is another name for white blood cell?

2. Which type of blood cell shows phagocytic properties?

3. What are the different kinds of white blood cells?

4. What do you call the needle used to make a finger puncture?

5. What do we call the liquid part of the blood?

6. What is another name for counting chamber?

7. In what piece of equipment is blood diluted before a count is taken?

8. What is the normal number of WBC/ml?

9. What is the normal number of RBC/ml?

10. What type of WBC is most numerous?

1. _____

2. _____

3. _____

4. _____

5. _____

6. _____

7. _____

8. _____

9. _____

10. _____

Answers

1. leukocyte
2. WBC (monocyte)
3. lymphocyte
   basophil
   neutrophil
   eosinophil
   monocyte
4. lancet
5. plasma
6. hemacytometer
7. Thoma pipette
8. 5000-10,000
9. 4½ million (women)
   5 million (men)
10. neutrophil

Problem **To study and count platelets.**

Background Information

Platelets are cells which are involved in the clotting of blood. They appear as small (1-5u) round or oval bluish bodies lying singly or in clumps. There are 200,000 to 300,000 per cc of blood.

Procedure

☐ 1. Draw a platelet solution into a RBC pipette.
☐ 2. Expel the solution from the pipette.
☐ 3. Make a finger puncture.
☐ 4. Draw blood to the 0.5 mark.
☐ 5. Draw the platelet solution to the 101 mark.
☐ 6. Mix the solution and the blood.
☐ 7. Fill the hemacytometer in the usual manner (discard the first few drops of blood).
☐ 8. Observe under LOW POWER.
☐ 9. Count the platelets in the 4 large corner squares used in making a white blood cell count.
   Platelets are not easy to see. They appear as small glistening bodies.
   Within each body there may be several platelets.
☐ 10. Multiply the number of cells by 2,000.
☐ 11. Complete this chart.

Chamber I	No. of platelets	Chamber II	No. of platelets
square 1 square 3 square 5 square 7			

total
average _____ x 2,000

Questions for Review

1. What is the function of platelets?
2. What may a deficiency of platelets indicate?

To learn to determine the amount of hemoglobin in the blood.

Lesson 12

Background Information

Hemoglobin is an iron containing protein present as a red pigment in the red blood cells. It carries oxygen to the cells of the body and carbon dioxide away from the cells. The amount of hemoglobin present in the blood cells depends on age and sex. A table shows normal ranges. Notice that the hemoglobin content is given in grams per ml of blood.

A lack of hemoglobin may indicate anemia (oligochromenia).

Group	Normal value g/100ml
infants at birth	18-27
childhood	10-15
adult males	14-17
adult females	12-16

Procedure

☐ 1. Remove a piece of absorbent paper from your *Tallquist* book.
☐ 2. Open the book to the last page. Notice a color chart, Tallquist scale, with a centrally located hole. Each color represents the color of blood. Each color indicates the percent of hemoglobin in the blood.
☐ 3. Make a finger puncture.
☐ 4. Blot a drop of blood with a piece of Tallquist paper (second drop of blood).
☐ 5. Allow the paper to dry until the sheen has disappeared.
☐ 6. Match the absorbent paper with the color of the Tallquist scale.
☐ 7. Record % of hemoglobin.

This method is one of the poorest used because there may be a 20-25% error, but it is the easiest. The best methods involve comparing the color of blood against a standard in electrically controlled machines.

Questions for Review

1. Why is the diagnosis of anemia important?
2. This method is not the best, but is the most often used. Explain.

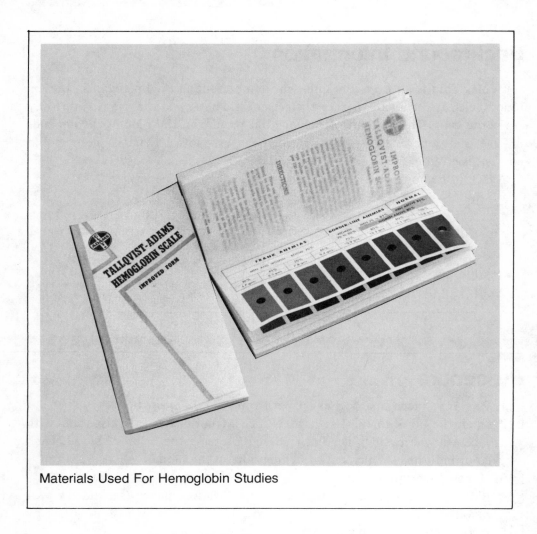

Materials Used For Hemoglobin Studies

To determine hemoglobin content by the use of the Sahli-Adams Method.

Lesson 13

Background Information

Hemoglobin may be removed from the RBC by using dilute HC1. The hemoglobin is converted to protein and acid hematin solution.

The Sahli-Adams method is similar to the comparative block indicator. The color of the tube containing hematin is matched to a brown-glass indicator. The amount of dilution needed to match the colors indicates the amount of hemoglobin present.

Procedure

☐ 1. Fill the graduated Hemometer tube to the 2gm mark (yellow) with dilute HC1. Use an eyedropper.

2 sides of Hemometer Tube

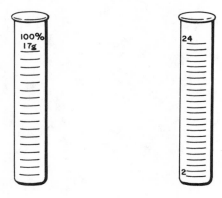

☐ 2. Draw blood into the pipette to the 20cc mark. A slight excess may be removed by touching the tip to a piece of cotton. If there is a large excess, discharge the pipette and begin again.

☐ 3. Wipe off excess blood from the outside of the pipette and place the tip well into the acid.
☐ 4. Slowly blow out the blood. Rinse the pipette by drawing the fluid in and out of the pipette several times. *Do not form air bubbles.* Blow gently through the pipette when removing it from the tube.
☐ 5. Mix the acid and blood with a stirring rod.
☐ 6. Allow to stand for 10 minutes.
☐ 7. Insert hemometer tube into hemometer.
☐ 8. Dilute the solution by adding distilled water a drop at a time until the color matches that of the standard brown glass. Stir after each drop.
☐ 9. Read the concentration of hemoglobin in grams per miligrams of blood from the scale on the hemometer (blue side). The meniscus of the acid hematin solution is the level read.
☐10. Compare the reading to the chart to obtain the percent.

Questions for Review

1. Which method is more accurate?
2. Which method is easiest to use?

Problem To study how to type blood.

Background Information

Red blood cells are cells which contain different kinds of proteins. It is recognized that not all red blood cells are alike; they have different properties depending on the proteins present. In addition the red blood cells are floating in a sea of plasma which in turn contains proteins. When blood of two different types is mixed, an antigen-antibody reaction occurs. The blood clots, agglutinates.

It was due to this observation that Dr. Landsteiner in 1900 developed a system for typing (classifying) blood. In his system there were 4 types of blood, A, B, O, and AB. What did this mean?

A person of type A blood has a RBC protein (agglutinogen) designated as A and a plasma protein (agglutinin) designated as b. The following chart may make this clearer.

type	RBC protein antigen (agglutinogen)	Plasma protein antibody (agglutinin)	
A	A	b	anti-B
B	B	a	anti-A
AB	AB	none	
O	none	a and b	anti-A, anti-B

Since blood of type A clots type B, each has a factor which works against (anti) the other. For the sake of ease, the factors were called anti-A and anti-B rather than a and b. This information makes blood typing an easy process. The serum or plasma of anti-A clots type A blood and the serum or plasma of anti-B clots type B blood.

Since Landsteiner's system of classification, other blood factors have been recognized. There are at least 45 different factors and many subdivisions to each blood type or group.

Lesson 14

Procedure

☐ 1. Divide a slide in half with a wax pencil.

☐ 2. Place the subject's initials or number in the lower right hand corner of the slide.

☐ 3. Label the upper left hand corner A.

☐ 4. Label the upper right hand corner B.

☐ 5. Place one drop of anti-B on the left side.

☐ 6. Place one drop of anti-A on the right side.

☐ 7. Make a finger puncture. Draw some blood into a pipette or allow a drop of blood to fall on each side of the slide into the serum.

☐ 8. Mix well for 5 to 10 seconds with a tooth pick. Allow to stand for 3 minutes.

☐ 9. Observe the slide for clumping.

If the blood on the A side clumps, the blood is type B.

If the blood on the B side clumps, the blood is type A.

If the blood on both sides clumps, the blood is type AB.

If the blood on neither side clumps, the blood is type O.

Type B

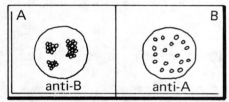

Type A

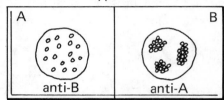

Type AB

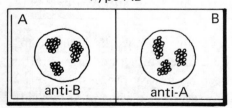

Type O

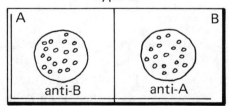

Questions for Review

1. Why is blood typing important?
2. What happens if a patient receives the wrong type of blood?
3. Can you determine the type of blood the donor must have to give to each recipient?

Recipient blood type	Donor
A	
B	
AB	
O	

4. Who is the universal donor?
5. Who is the universal recipient?

Problem

To study how to determine the Rh factor of the blood.

Lesson 15

Background Information

Rabbits were injected with the RBC from the Rhesus monkey by Landsteiner and Wiener. As expected the Rhesus RBC were destroyed. When the serum from the rabbits was added to human RBC, 85% of the samples clumped. Before the rabbit serum had been treated with Rhesus RBC, no such action occurred. It was concluded that the RBC of the Rhesus monkey caused the rabbit serum to develop antibodies. These antibodies were able to attack the RBC of the human. This meant that the human RBC contained the same protein that the Rhesus monkey had. 85% of the people had the Rhesus protein (factor) and were designated Rh+ while the other 15% that did not have the factor were designated Rh-.

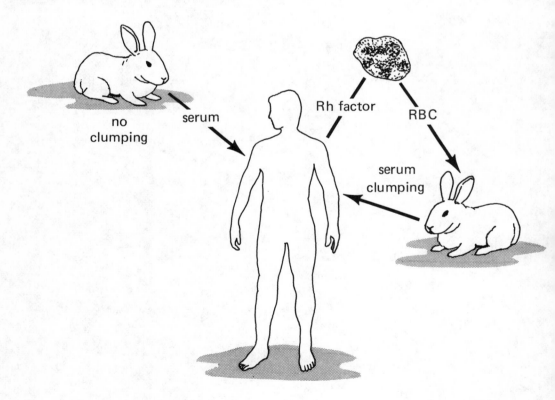

no clumping   serum   Rh factor   RBC   serum clumping

Laboratory Techniques

What was the significance of this discovery? The Rh factor explained why people who received properly typed transfusions developed complications and why children were born with a fatal disease, erythroblastosis fetalis.

The Rh factor is genetically controlled. The gene for Rh+ is dominant over the Rh- gene. If a negative woman marries a positive man, the child will be positive. The mother's blood stream will develop antibodies to counteract the presence of the child's Rh+ factor. These antibodies can destroy the child's RBC. However, this situation may not arise until the third pregnancy when there is a tremendous amount of antibodies in the mother's blood stream.

Procedure

☐ 1. Place one drop of anti-Rh serum on a preheated slide. Heat over microscope lamp.
☐ 2. Make a finger puncture. Discard first drop of blood.
☐ 3. Place one drop of blood in the serum.
☐ 4. Mix with a tooth pick.
☐ 5. Observe after 2 minutes.
   If the blood cells clump, label Rh+.
   If the blood cells do not clump, label Rh-.

Questions for Review

1. Why is it necessary to type for the Rh factor?
2. Determine the possible Rh factor of the offspring resulting from each marriage.

Lesson 15

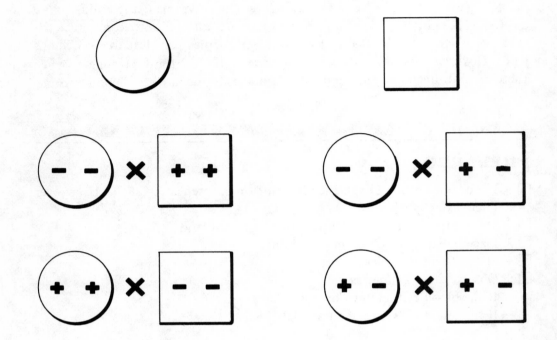

To study bleeding time.

Background Information

The bleeding time is the time it takes for a wound to stop bleeding. The stopping of the flow of blood from an injured part of the body is called hemostasis. Hemostasis is brought about by the proper action of blood vessel walls and the chemical activity of the blood itself. Any defect in this mechanism indicates a disease. Bleeding time is primarily concerned with the operation of injured blood vessels.

Procedure

☐ 1. Make a finger puncture. In order to insure a standard sized puncture, one person in the group should make the puncture.
Note the time that the first drop of blood appeared. _____
☐ 2. Blot drop with filter paper every 10 seconds. Only the top of the drop should be touched with the paper.
☐ 3. Continue this procedure until no drops appear.
☐ 4. Record the time of the last drop. _____
☐ 5. The time between the puncture and the last drop is considered the bleeding time.
The normal time is 1 to 3 minutes.

Question for Review

1. Why is it important to know bleeding time?

Problem To study coagulation time.

Background Information

The coagulation time is the interval of time needed for the blood to form a clot, the time it takes for the fibrin fibers to appear. Clotting depends on the chemical activity of the blood itself. The actual clotting mechanism is very complex and involves many steps. However, it can be summarized.

The damaged or punctured tissues release fluids which attract and rupture platelets. The ruptured platelets release a substance, thrombokinase, which allows calcium and prothrombin, a plasma protein, to combine to form thrombin. This immediately combines with fibrinogen, another plasma protein, to form fibrin. The strands of fibrin form a mesh which traps red blood cells and seals the wound. This entire process takes between 3 to 5 minutes. In diseases such as hemophilia there are no platelets and a person can bleed to death from a pin prick.

Procedure

☐ 1. Make a deep finger puncture.
☐ 2. Allow the first 2 drops of blood to flow then fill 5 or 6 capillary tubes ¾ of the way. Note the time you began to fill the first tube. _____
☐ 3. Seal the ends of the capillary tubes.
☐ 4. Every 30 seconds tilt the tubes until the blood no longer flows.
☐ 5. Break off a small segment of the tube every 30 seconds until a fibrin thread connects the 2 broken ends of the tube. Note the time. _____

Question for Review

1. Why is it important to know the coagulation time?

To determine RBC Sedimentation Rate (ESR).

Background Information

If blood is allowed to stand in a test tube after an anticoagulant is added, the RBC will settle out. Because the cells are heavy, they fall to the bottom leaving the clear plasma at the top. The anticoagulant is added to prevent a clot from forming. Clots prevent the separation of cells from the plasma. Under normal conditions the cells fall at a specific rate.

Sedimentation Rate	Men	Women
Normal	1-6 mm/hr	1-9 mm/hr
Slightly high	7-15 mm/hr	10-15 mm/hr
Moderately high	16-30 mm/hr	16-30 mm/hr
High	Over 30 mm/hr	Over 30 mm/hr

If there has been tissue damage caused by disease, there is an increase in fibrinogen or globulin. The presence of abnormal amounts of these proteins increases the sedimentation rate. (In cases of tuberculosis, cancer, rheumatic fever, rheumatoid arthritis, and anemia, the sedimentation rate is high.) This test cannot be used to diagnose a specific disease, but it is used to suggest that a disease condition exists.

Procedure

☐ 1. Draw a 5% sodium citrate solution to the first or lowest mark on the sedimentation pipette.

☐ 2. Make a finger puncture. Discard the first drop of blood.

☐ 3. Draw the blood until it reaches the upper mark on the pipette.

☐ 4. Draw the blood into the bulb, but not completely. The lower meniscus should be a few millimeters from the bulb.

☐ 5. Force the blood down into the sedimentation pipette.

☐ 6. Follow procedure 4 and 5 two more times. This allows the blood to mix with the sodium citrate solution.

☐ 7. Insert the pipette in its holder.

☐ 8. After one hour, record the reading. Each line on the pipette is graduated in millimeters.

Lesson 18

Questions for Review

1. Why is this test not used as a diagnostic test?
2. Why bother to perform this test if it does not tell us what disease is present?

Hematology Summary Sheet

No. RBC _____

% hemoglobin _____

No. WBC _____

Differential count _____

    neutrophils _____

    eosinophils _____

    monocytes _____

    lymphocytes _____

    basophils _____

Platelet count _____

Bleeding time _____

Coagulation time _____

Blood Type _____

Rh factor _____

Lesson 18

TEST YOURSELF

1. What type of blood cell is necessary for clotting?

    1. _____

2. What is another name for the bleeder's disease?

    2. _____

3. What is the colored protein found in the RBC?

    3. _____

4. Which is the easiest method for determining hemoglobin percent?

    4. _____

5. What disease is associated with small amounts of hemoglobin?

    5. _____

6. What type blood does the universal donor have?

    6. _____

7. What type blood does a universal recipient have?

    7. _____

8. What blood factor is involved in "blue babies"?

    8. _____

9. What is the normal bleeding time?

    9. _____

10. What is the normal coagulation time?

    10. _____

Answers

1. platelet
2. hemophilia
3. hemoglobin
4. Tallquist
5. anemia
6. O
7. AB
8. Rh
9. 1-3 minutes
10. 3-5 minutes

Glossary

ABO system   A system of classifying (typing) blood.

amoeboid   Having the movement of an amoeba.

agglutinin   A protein found in RBC.

agglutinogen   A protein found in the plasma.

antibody   A chemical substance produced by the body to combat antigens.

antigen   A foreign protein or organism.

differential count   A counting of the different types of WBC on a stained smear.

Hayems solution   A fluid used to destroy WBC and dilute RBC for a count.

hemacytometer   A blood cell counting chamber.

hemoglobin   A red pigment in the RBC which carries oxygen.

lancet   A needle used to make a finger puncture.

leukocyte   Another name for WBC.

phagocytic   Having the ability to take in microorganisms.

plasma   The liquid part of the blood.

platelet   A type of blood cell necessary for blood clotting.

serum   The liquid part of the blood which is free from fibrinogen.

Thoma pipette   A pipette used for diluting blood.

Wright's stain   A stain used to distinguish the different types of blood cell by giving them color.

Unit III

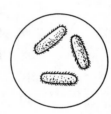

Bacteriology

Unit III Table of Contents

Bacteriology

Many times you hear T.V. commercials advertising products that "kill germs." The word, germ, implies bacteria. Although some bacteria are pathogenic (disease causing) there are many non-pathogens. Several species of bacteria are useful in the manufacture of important industrial products (cheese, beer, wine, rope). Others are useful for natural events. Nitrates could not be restored to the soil if the nitrifying, dentrifying and nitrogen fixing bacteria did not do their work. Bacteria of decay are useful to man also.

Bacteria are single celled organisms which have a cell wall composed of cellulose. Because of this feature they were traditionally classified as plants. However, they are not green, photosynthetic plants. They are currently classified as Protista. Bacteria lack an organized nucleus. There are special features which bacteria may have such as flagella (whip-like structures), slime capsules, and pili.

In general, bacteria are classified according to shape. Bacillus is rod shaped. Coccus is a round bacterium. Spirillum has a spiral shape. However, species of bacteria vary in the environmental needs, temperature requirements, places of growth, and metabolic activity. Because of these differences they can be identified.

Identification of the pathogenic bacteria is extremely important for the prevention of disease epidemics and the maintenance of good health. The following procedures are designed to familiarize the student with some of the techniques employed in identification. Since bacteriology may be dangerous, only non-pathogens will be used in the high school laboratory.

A GENERALIZED BACTERIAL CELL

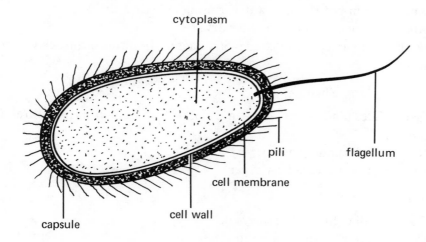

cytoplasm

pili

flagellum

cell membrane

cell wall

capsule

Problem To learn how to clean glassware for bacterial studies .

Background Information

Before you begin the study of bacteria, you should become familiar with cleaning procedures which must be followed. All glassware should be free from particles before use. The slightest contamination will interfere with the growth of the bacteria. You will be handling microscopic organisms which must be removed from the glassware when you no longer need them.

YOUR TABLE MUST BE WASHED WITH LYSOL BEFORE AND AFTER EACH LABORATORY PERIOD.

Procedure

Glassware

☐1. Place glassware in hot water, add enough soap to make plenty of suds.
☐2. Scrub well with a brush.
☐3. Rinse well in hot running water, rinsing at least 3 times.
☐4. Allow glassware to drain and air dry.
☐5. If glassware is contaminated with bacterial cultures, autoclave and then wash.

Slides and Cover Slips

☐1. Place slides and cover slips in lysol. Then boil in soapy water for 10 minutes.
☐2. Rinse in hot running water.
☐3. Drain and polish (use lens paper).

Pipettes

☐1. Place in tall cylinder full of lysol.
☐2. Use the water suction pump to clean.
☐3. Sterilize.

Questions for Review

1. Why must all the soap be removed from the glassware?
2. Why must you clean the tables before and after each period?

Problem	# To study how to sterilize equipment.

Background Information

There are many kinds of bacteria present in the air. All equipment used to culture bacteria should be free from unwanted bacteria. In order to obtain sterile equipment, an *autoclave* will be used. The autoclave is a pressure cooker. The water at the bottom is converted to steam by the heat from a burner. The steam is not allowed to escape and pressure is built up. The steam under pressure kills most bacteria.

Procedure

☐1. Place clean glassware into the autoclave.
☐2. Steam for 15-20 minutes at 15-20 pounds of pressure (121°C).
☐3. Allow autoclave to cool.
☐4. Remove, use, or store sterile equipment.

Autoclave Procedures

☐1. Open valve so that the steam can escape.
☐2. When the steam begins to escape, close the valve.
☐3. If the pressure gauge goes above the desired value, open the valve slightly or lower the flame.
☐4. When sterilization is completed, allow the autoclave to cool.
☐5. Open and remove equipment.

Questions for Review

1. Why must glassware be clean before sterilization?
2. A student trying to grow type A bacteria finds type B and type C also growing in the same Petri dish. Explain.

Growth Requirements

All bacteria require food for growth. Some are autotrophic (can produce their own food) but the heterotrophic organisms have been studied the most. While some bacteria grow best on specific substances, common food sources such as beef extracts, peptone, and yeast extracts will allow most bacteria to grow. Agar, a carbohydrate obtained from a specific marine algae, is added to the extracts to solidify the medium. Agar itself is not a nutrient source. If you read the labels of the commercially prepared nutrient agar, you will note that other substances have been added. You may purchase pure agar and add different nutrients to it according to the needs of your experiment.

Nutrient broth is basically composed of the same food materials as nutrient agar. But the agar is lacking. It is sometimes best to cultivate the organisms in a liquid medium depending upon what you are testing for. In addition there are different kinds of agar and broths (EMB, dextrose, lactose, etc.).

Most of the bacteria studied in class will grow at temperatures of 25° C to 40° C. The temperature at which the organism grows best is the optimum temperature. It varies according to the organism. You will notice that some of the organisms grown in class require more time to grow than others. One of the factors influencing this is the lack of control of the temperature in the classroom.

Some bacteria require oxygen for growth (aerobes) while others grow in the absence of oxygen (anaerobes). Still others can grow in either condition (facultative anaerobes). Most of the organisms grown in class are aerobic. Because of this, streak plates must be properly prepared if you wish to observe growth over a 24 hr. period. Improper preparation will curtail growth.

For successful culturing (growing bacteria under laboratory conditions) all their growth requirements should be considered.

To study how to prepare broth.

Background Information

In order for bacteria to grow they need food, moisture, and heat. Liquid broth (soup) is often used as a medium (food). There are different kinds of broths.

Procedure

☐ 1. Follow the directions accompanying the jar of broth.
☐ 2. Pour into test tubes - Fill 2/3.
☐ 3. Plug.
☐ 4. Sterilize at 15 pounds of pressure for 15-20 minutes.
☐ 5. Store in refrigerator until needed.

Questions for Review

1. What is a nutrient broth?
2. When would you use nutrient broth?

Problem # To prepare agar tubes.

Background Information

In order to study bacteria, you may have to grow them on a solid medium. Nutrient agar contains most of the substances that bacteria need to grow.

Procedure

☐ 1. Follow the directions which accompany the agar.
☐ 2. Pour liquid agar into a large beaker.
☐ 3. Place beaker in a water bath. Stir until all the agar is dissolved and the solution appears clear.
☐ 4. Place a funnel that is slightly warm on a ring stand.
☐ 5. When the agar is cool enough to handle, pour through the funnel into test tubes.
☐ 6. Fill the tubes half way. You must work quickly to prevent the agar from hardening.
☐ 7. Allow the agar tubes to cool, then cap.
☐ 8. Sterilize the tubes at 15 pounds of pressure for 15-20 minutes.
☐ 9. Place ½ of the test tubes in a slanted position—agar slants.
☐10. Refrigerate hardened agar until needed.

Questions for Review

1. Why is sterilization important?
2. What is the difference between agar slants and agar tubes?

Growth and Reproduction

When the term growth is used for bacterial organisms, it does not imply growth of individual cells, but an increase in the entire population of cells. Therefore, growth means reproduction.

Reproduction occurs asexually (one individual). It involves a process called binary fission (transverse splitting). There is also sexual reproduction observed in some bacteria (conjugation). In this case chromosomal material passes from one cell to another by crossing over a cytoplasmic bridge formed between two cells. Strictly speaking, this process allows for genetic variation, and is not the primary means of increasing in numbers.

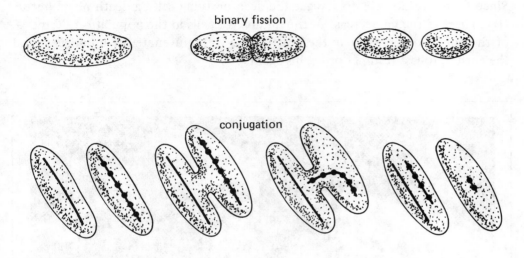

The time it takes for the population to double is called the generation time. This varies with the kinds of bacteria and the growing conditions (temperature, medium). The growth of the bacteria can be plotted on a curve.

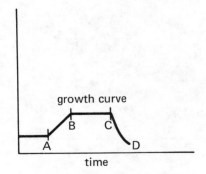

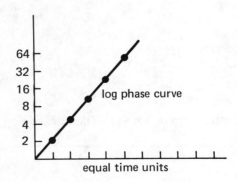

Lesson 4

During (A) the lag phase, the cells are increasing in size and preparing for division. This is the phase in which no growth is revealed.

During (B) the log phase, the cells divide. The increase is seen as a straight line. One cell becomes 2, 2 becomes 4, 4 becomes 8, 8 becomes 16, etc. Cell division occurs during equal time units.

Growth eventually ceases due to many factors. The nutritive material may be consumed or waste products inhibit growth. The population remains constant for a certain time, the stationary phase (C).

Because of unfavorable environmental conditions, cells stop reproducing. Since there are no cells to replace the dead or dying cells, a death phase occurs (D). There is then a decrease in the number of cells in the population. Removal of the conditions present in the death phase will rejuvenate the population and the entire process resumes or begins again.

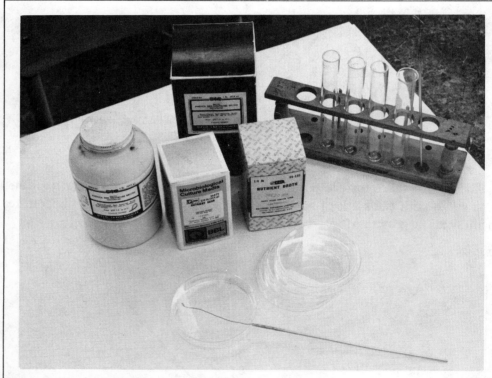

Some Materials Used In The Bacteriology Laboratory

Laboratory Techniques

Lesson 4

TEST YOURSELF

1. How many types of bacteria are there?
2. Which cell structure allows an organism to move?
3. What do we call organisms that cause disease?
4. What apparatus is used to sterilize equipment?
5. Growing bacteria under laboratory conditions is called
6. The nutritive substance used in culturing is called
7. What material do aerobes require for growth?
8. What is a solid medium called?
9. Bacteria reproduce asexually by a process called
10. Bacteria reproduce sexually by a process called

1. _____
2. _____
3. _____
4. _____
5. _____
6. _____
7. _____
8. _____
9. _____
10. _____

Answers

1. three
2. flagellum
3. pathogens
4. autoclave
5. culturing
6. medium
7. oxygen
8. agar-agar
9. binary fission
10. conjugation

Staining

In the lessons that follow, you will learn how to stain bacteria. There are two types of stains, the simple and the differential stain. Some special stains, such as the acid-fast and spore stain, are also used. Why do bacterial organisms pick up the various stains?

Most bacteria contain acid (nucleic acid) within their cells. The acid is easily neutralized by a basic dye resulting in a salt formation. Methylene blue, crystal violet, and many other stains are basic. When a bacterial cell becomes visible, it is because of the salt crystals within it.

A differential stain, Gram stain, is not only tricky to do, but also may be difficult to understand. This stain employs two dyes, crystal violet (blue) and safranin (red). If the bacteria retain the blue dye, they are Gram positive. If they retain the pink stain, they are Gram negative. The dye which the bacteria retain depends upon the composition of the cell wall and the amount of RNA present. Crystal violet combines with the RNA (nucleic acid). When iodine is added, the union becomes permanent. The cell wall of Gram + bacteria is composed of 2-4% lipids (fats). Alcohol which is used to decolorize the cell causes the cell wall to dehydrate and become very compact. This prevents the dye from being washed out.

Gram - bacteria have 1/8 as much RNA which means that less salt is formed. The cell wall contains 15% lipids making dehydration less pronounced. The wall does not become very compact, instead it becomes porous. When the cells are washed, the crystal violet is also washed out. The counter-stain is then easily picked up.

What is the significance of the Gram stain? Most organisms are either + or -. Identification makes treatment possible. Gram + organisms are extremely susceptible to penicillin while Gram - organisms are susceptible to streptomycin. Gram + organisms release metabolic wastes into the blood stream (exotoxins) which poison the individual, while Gram - organisms produce endotoxins. These poisons are released only when the organism disintegrates. Exotoxin producing organisms are more virulent than the endotoxin producing organisms. Virulence refers to the capacity of an organism to produce a disease. Tetanus, pneumonia, botulism, diphtheria, and many other diseases are caused by Gram + organisms. In addition, there are some organisms that are Gram variable, that is, they may be + or - depending upon their environment, while others may be Gram - but behave like Gram + *(Neisseria gonorrhea)*. Other special tests are then necessary to identify these organisms.

To study how to prepare a slide for staining (film or smear).

Problem

Background Information

When you examine bacteria under the microscope, they are the same color as the broth in which they are living (colorless). In order to make bacteria visible, stains or dyes are used. Before a stain can be used, the bacteria must be fixed on a slide.

Procedure

☐ 1. Polish a clean glass slide with lens paper.
☐ 2. Draw a circle with a glass marking pencil in the center of the slide.
☐ 3. Turn the slide upside down so that the pencil mark rests on the desk.
☐ 4. Flame wire loop until it is white hot.
☐ 5. Remove the cap from the culture tube and hold it in your hand so that it does not become contaminated.
☐ 6. Flame the mouth of the culture tube.
☐ 7. Insert the wire loop into the culture tube. You should hear a sizzling sound.
☐ 8. Swish the loop gently in the broth and remove it without touching the sides of the test tube.
☐ 9. Touch the loop to the slide within the circular area.
☐ 10. Spread the material with the loop.
☐ 11. Flame the mouth of the tube and cap.
☐ 12. Flame the loop.
☐ 13. Allow the slide to air dry. Do not blow on it.
☐ 14. When the slide is dried, pass it through the flame 2 or 3 times. This *fixes*, kills and makes the bacteria stick to the slide.
☐ 15. Prepare smears for each bacteria. Make sure to label a corner of the slide with the name of the organism.

Lesson 5

Questions for Review

1. Why must the wire loop be flamed?
2. Why is the mouth of the culture tube flamed?
3. Why is the air dried slide passed through the flame?
4. What do you mean by fixing bacteria?
5. What will happen if you do not flame the loop or culture tube?

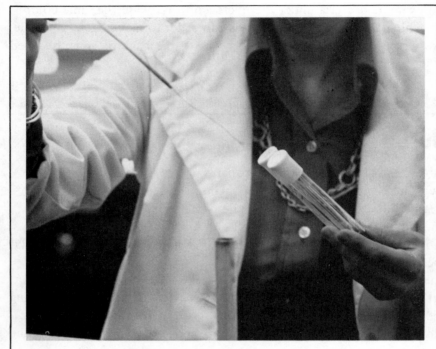

Method Of Holding Culture Tubes And Wire Inoculating Loop.

To study how to stain a slide with a simple stain.

Lesson 6

Background Information

In order to make bacteria visible under the microscope, you must stain them. A simple stain is just one stain which makes the bacteria stand out. Methylene blue, safranin, carbol fuchsin, and Bismark brown are simple stains. We will use *methylene blue*.

Procedure

☐ 1. Make a film.
☐ 2. Place the slide, film side up, on a staining tray.
☐ 3. Flood the slide with methylene blue for 1½ minutes.
☐ 4. Wash the slide with water.
☐ 5. With the film side down, blot the slide dry between 2 layers of paper toweling. Do not rub.
☐ 6. Examine under HP or oil immersion.
☐ 7. Complete this chart.

organism	shape	size
1.		
2.		
3.		
4.		
5.		

☐ 8. Make a diagram of each organism.

Questions for Review

1. What procedures did you follow to prevent contamination of the culture?
2. What differences do you notice among the cells?

Problem To study differential staining techniques.

Background Information

Differential staining involves the use of several stains. This technique shows the differences between different kinds of bacteria and different cell structures.

The Gram stain allows us to divide bacteria into two groups, Gram + and Gram -. The Gram + bacteria appear violet or blue in color and the Gram - appear red to pink in color. These two types are different in their susceptibility to drugs. By identifying bacteria as + or -, a diagnosis and treatment can be made easier.

Procedure

☐ 1. Make a smear.
☐ 2. Flood the fixed, cooled smear with Gram's crystal violet stain for 1½ minutes. Be sure the slide is on the staining tray.
☐ 3. Pour off the dye and wash slide with water.
☐ 4. Flood the slide with Gram's iodine for one minute. Iodine is a mordant, it fixes the Gram + cells so that they will not lose the violet color.
☐ 5. Pour off the iodine and wash. Decolorize the slide with 95% ethyl alcohol. Add the alcohol a drop at a time until the material running off the slide is colorless.
☐ 6. Remove the alcohol at once by washing in cold water.
☐ 7. Flood the slide with safranin for 1½ minutes.
☐ 8. Pour off safranin, wash slide, blot dry.
☐ 9. Examine slide. Complete chart.

organism	Gram stain
1.	
2.	
3.	
4.	

If the bacteria are blue or violet, they are Gram +.
If the bacteria are red or pink, they are Gram -.

Question for Review

1. What advantage is differential staining over simple staining?

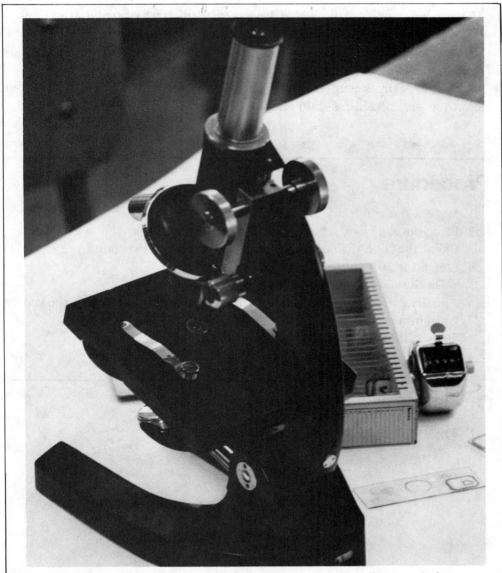

The Microscope, Slides, Slide Box And Counter Are Used Frequently In
The Medical Laboratory.

Problem # To study acid-fast bacteria.

Background Information

There are some bacteria which have a very thick waxy material in their cell walls. They do not take the Gram stain easily, although they are considered Gram positive. These organisms belong to the group *Mycobacterium*. Some of them are the cause of tuberculosis and leprosy.

A special stain is used to identify these organisms. It is called the acid-fast stain. Acid-fast organisms stain red while non-acid fast organisms stain blue.

Procedure

☐1. Make a smear (air dry and fix).
☐2. Place the slide over a beaker of boiling water.
☐3. Flood the slide with carbol fuchsin. Do not allow the stain to dry.
☐4. Steam for 10 minutes.
☐5. Wash the slide in water.
☐6. Add acid alcohol a drop at a time until no more color runs off the slide.
☐7. Wash in water.
☐8. Stain with methylene blue for 1 minute.
☐9. Wash in water and blot dry.

Question for Review

1. Why is this procedure important?

To make a spore stain (Dorner Method).

Background Information

At some point in the life cycle of some bacteria, a hard outer covering may develop within the cell wall. Water is lost and the cytoplasmic material shrinks forming a *spore*. Many bacilli are spore formers. The hard outer case makes it difficult to destroy the bacteria.

The size, shape, and position of the spore within the cell differs with each kind of bacteria. Because of this, it is sometimes possible to identify bacteria on the basis of their spores.

Procedure

☐ 1. Make a smear (air dry and fix).
☐ 2. Add 5% chromic acid for 2 minutes (flood slide).
☐ 3. Wash the slide with water.
☐ 4. Place the slide over a beaker of boiling water for 10 minutes. This softens the spore wall and allows the stain to enter.
☐ 5. Flood the slide with carbol fuchsin. Do not allow the stain to dry on the slide. This procedure is combined with step 4.
☐ 6. Wash the slide in water.
☐ 7. Add alcohol a drop at a time until the stain appears light pink.
☐ 8. Wash in water.
☐ 9. Add methylene blue for 1 minute.
☐ 10. Observe. The spore will appear pink and the surrounding cell blue.

Questions for Review

1. Why is an old culture of bacteria used?
2. Which bacteria produce spores?

Lesson 9

TEST YOURSELF

Staining

1. What dye is used most often in simple staining?

2. What is the mordant in the Gram stain?

3. What drugs are Gram + organisms most susceptible to?

4. Toxins released by living organisms are called

5. Toxins released by dead organisms are called

6. What substance in the bacterial cell wall is responsible for the degree of dehydration?

7. Which group of bacteria are acid-fast?

8. What type of bacteria form spores?

9. What is the process called which allows bacteria to stick to a slide after they have been killed?

10. What color are Gram - bacteria stained?

1. _____

2. _____

3. _____

4. _____

5. _____

6. _____

7. _____

8. _____

9. _____

10. _____

Answers

1. methylene blue
2. iodine
3. penicillin
4. exotoxins
5. endotoxins
6. lipids
7. Mycobacterium
8. bacillus
9. fixing
10. red-pink

To study living bacteria in a hanging-drop.

Problem

Lesson 10

Background Information

In order to examine bacteria, two methods can be used; organisms may be suspended in a liquid-hanging drop or they may be prepared as a smear.

The hanging-drop method is used to study living bacteria. This method removes most of the distortion that results when you prepare a smear. It also allows you to see if the bacteria are motile (can move). If they are motile, they must have at least one flagellum.

Procedure

☐ 1. Using a tooth pick, put a little vaseline around the depression of a special hanging-drop slide (depression slide).

☐ 2. Place a cover slip flat on the table.

☐ 3. With the wire loop, place one drop of fluid from the culture broth in the center of the cover slip.

☐ 4. Invert the slide (hole facing table) and place it directly on top of the cover slip so that the drop is directly in the center.

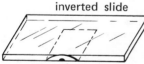
inverted slide
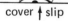
cover ↑ slip

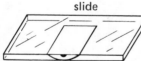
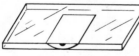
slide

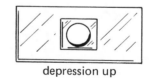
depression up

☐ 5. Press slide gently to make a perfect seal.

☐ 6. Invert the slide so that the cover slip now faces the ceiling.

☐ 7. Examine under LP to find the drop. Focus on the edge. REDUCE LIGHT.

☐ 8. Turn to HP and examine. If the organisms are motile, they move in a particular direction. Motion which is back and forth and haphazard is called *Brownian movement*. An organism showing Brownian movement does not move by itself and is *non-motile*.

☐ 9. Complete this chart.

organism	motility
1.	
2.	
3.	
4.	

Questions for Review

1. Why is it important to determine motility?
2. What procedures are followed to prevent contamination of the culture?

To study how to transfer bacteria into agar slants.

Lesson 11

Background Information

It is necessary to grow one kind of bacterium at a time (pure culture). In order to maintain this type of culture, we must transfer bacteria from one medium to another. The agar slants are best used to maintain a culture since they provide a wide surface area for growth. In the transfer process care is taken as not to contaminate the culture.

Procedure

☐ 1. Hold both test tubes in a slanted position to prevent dust from entering.
☐ 2. Flame wire loop.
☐ 3. Remove caps. Hold the caps between the 3rd and 4th fingers of one hand so that they do not touch anything.
☐ 4. Pass both test tubes through the flame.
☐ 5. Insert sterile loop into test tube containing bacteria.
☐ 6. Remove loop. Bacteria may not appear to be on the loop. Remember that they are microscopic.
☐ 7. Stroke the surface of the slant with the loop. Cover the entire surface but do not break or cut into the surface.
☐ 8. Pass mouth of both tubes through flame.
☐ 9. Recap both tubes.
☐10. Flame loop.
☐11. Label the newly inoculated tube with the name of the bacteria and date of transfer.
☐12. Incubation. Most bacteria require a certain temperature to grow. To insure growth, cultures are placed in an incubator which maintains a constant temperature. The best temperature is $35°C-36°C$. The time required for growth depends on the bacteria.

Questions for Review

1. Why should the caps be held in such a way as not to touch anything?
2. Why are the mouths of the tubes passed through a flame?
3. Why is the loop flamed before and after it is inserted into the culture tube?

Lesson 12

Problem

To study the pattern of growth of bacteria on agar slants.

Background Information

Each species of bacteria grows in a special manner or pattern on agar slants. The pattern may be helpful in identification of the bacteria.

Procedure

☐1. Examine the agar slants — do not remove caps.
☐2. Compare the type of growth with a special sheet.
☐3. Complete this chart.

organism	pattern of growth
1.	
2.	
3.	
4.	

Question for Review

1. How can the growth pattern of bacteria be useful?

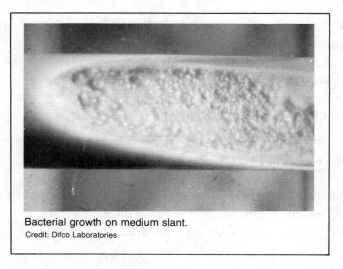

Bacterial growth on medium slant.
Credit: Difco Laboratories

Problem

To study how to make a streak plate.

Lesson 13

Background Information

A streak plate is used to separate bacterial cells from each other so that each bacterium can grow and reproduce forming a colony. The colonies are separated from each other so that you can study them easily.

Procedure

- ☐ 1. Flame wire loop.
- ☐ 2. Uncap culture tube.
- ☐ 3. Flame mouth of tube.
- ☐ 4. Place loop into culture tube and remove a loopful of material—*inoculum*.
- ☐ 5. Flame mouth of tube and recap.
- ☐ 6. Open Petri dish slightly.
- ☐ 7. Touch the loop to one spot in the Petri dish and spread the inoculum across ¼ of the area.
- ☐ 8. Remove loop and reflame.
- ☐ 9. Touch loop to the portion of agar not inoculated.
- ☐10. Touch the loop to the streaked area and carry the inoculum out at right angles to the first streak.
- ☐11. Remove loop and reflame.
- ☐12. Touch loop to the second streak and carry the inoculum into the sterile agar at right angles to the second streak.

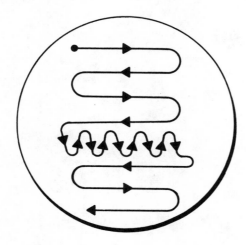

Fig. 5

Lesson 13

Questions for Review

1. What procedures are followed to avoid contamination?
2. Why do you not remove the entire cover of the Petri dish?
3. Why should each streaked section show less bacterial growth?

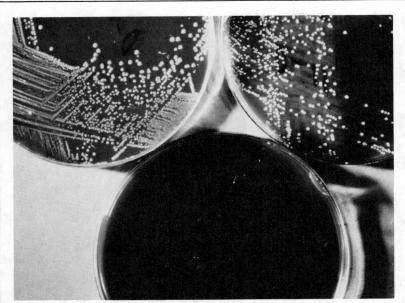

Typical colonies of intestinal bacteria growing on Brilliant Green Agar.
The plate at the bottom is uninoculated.
The plate at the upper right shows colonies of *E. coli*.
The plate at the upper left shows Salmonella colonies.
Credit: Difco Laboratories

To study the characteristics of colonial growth in agar plates.

Lesson 14

Background Information

Each kind of bacteria grows in a unique colonial form. A colony is a group of bacteria which came from the reproduction of one single bacterial cell.

Procedure

☐1. With a magnifying glass, examine the edge of one colony.
☐2. Compare the type of edge to the sheet.
☐3. Examine several colonies in the plate. They should all be of the same type of edging.
☐4. Complete this chart.

organism	type of colony
1.	
2.	
3.	
4.	

Question for Review

1. How is this procedure similar to agar slant examination?

To study characteristics of growth in a broth culture.

Problem

Background Information

Bacteria grow in different patterns depending on the type. The pattern of growth can be useful in identifying the type of bacteria.

Procedure

- ☐ 1. Hold the culture tube and broth in one hand so that you can see into both tubes.
- ☐ 2. Flame loop.
- ☐ 3. Remove caps from both tubes.
- ☐ 4. Flame mouth of both tubes.
- ☐ 5. Insert loop into culture.
- ☐ 6. Remove loop and insert into broth.
- ☐ 7. Flame mouth of both tubes and recap.
- ☐ 8. Flame loop.
- ☐ 9. Label broth with name of organism and date of transfer.
- ☐ 10. Incubate.

Patterns of Growth

PELLICLE - bacteria may grow only on the top and form a layer. This layer may or may not be colored.

TURBID - bacteria may grow evenly throughout the broth making it cloudy.

SEDIMENT - bacteria may grow only on the bottom forming a clump.

COMBINATION - of all three types may be found.

- ☐ 11. Complete this chart.

organism	growth pattern
1.	
2.	
3.	
4.	

Questions for Review

1. What procedures are used to prevent contamination of the culture and broth tubes?
2. What is the purpose of incubation?
3. Why should a label be dated?

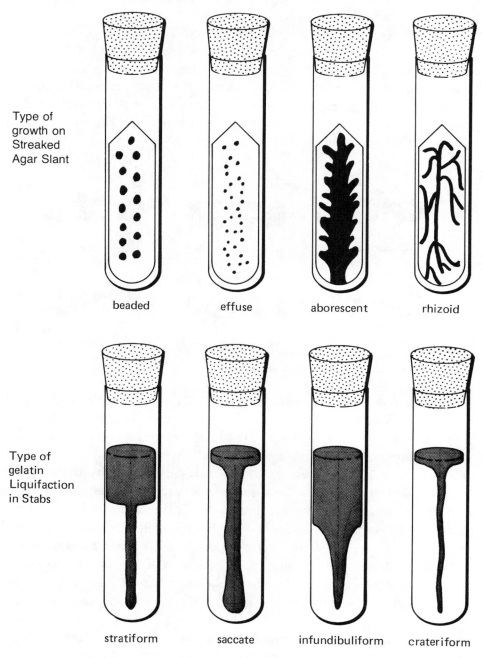

Type of growth on Streaked Agar Slant

| beaded | effuse | aborescent | rhizoid |

Type of gelatin Liquifaction in Stabs

| stratiform | saccate | infundibuliform | crateriform |

Types of colonies found on Agar Plates

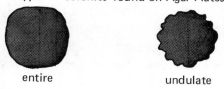

| entire | undulate |

Enzymes

Enzymes are complex protein molecules which speed up chemical reactions. For each chemical reaction, there is a specific enzyme. It is estimated that there must be about 2,000 different enzymes in a single animal cell. However, only small quantities of each are needed. Since enzymes are not used up in a chemical reaction, they can be reused.

Enzymes operate on a *lock and key* theory. The enzyme is the key which opens the lock (chemical reaction). If you examine keys carefully, you will notice that the teeth are different. Enzymes are different in shape due to the different arrangement of their atoms. Their teeth may be considered the *active sites* or the points where the enzymes couple with the chemical substances (substrate). After the enzyme has either opened or closed the lock (substrate), it is free to continue its work.

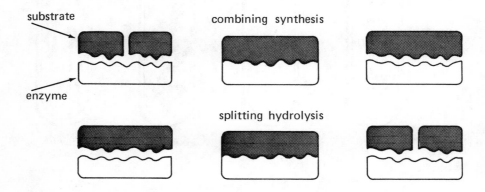

Certain enzymes work best under specific pH and temperature. A change in any of these conditions may inactivate the enzyme. Substances which tie up the active sites by permanently combining with them are called poisons. Cyanides, florides, and arsenics are poisons.

Fermentation is the process by which energy is released by the break down of carbohydrates (sugars) in the absence of oxygen. The energy is utilized by the bacteria to carry on its life processes. Enzymes are necessary for this process. In the fermentation process, sugars are split into acid and gas. The acids may be acetic, propionic, lactic, or succinic, while the gases may be CO_2 or H_2. In addition, alcohols may be produced, ethyl or butyl alcohol. Since there are different sugars, there must be different enzymes for each. If bacteria lack the specific enzymes necessary to split the sugars, there will be no fermentation.

Starch is composed of hundreds of sugar units joined together. Some bacteria have the enzymes necessary to split starch into their component sugars, which can then be used by the organism as a source of energy.

The *proteins* found in the medium in which bacteria are growing are too complex to enter the cell. They must be broken down into amino acids. In order to do this, enzymes must be present. Gelatin is the protein often used to test an organism's hydrolyzing (protein enzyme) activity.

One of the toxic materials produced by cells is H_2O_2, hydrogen peroxide. This substance is broken down to water and oxygen.

$$2H_2O_2 \text{------------} \longrightarrow 2H_2O \ + \ O_2$$

The ability of microorganisms to carry out this reaction depends on the presence of *catalase* (enzyme).

Some organisms can change nitrates to nitrites while others go one step further by changing nitrites to ammonia.

$$H^+ \ + \ NaNO_3 \text{------} \blacktriangleright NaNO_2 \ + \ H_2O$$
$$\text{nitrate} \qquad\qquad \text{nitrite} \qquad \text{water}$$
$$NaNO_2 \text{------} \blacktriangleright NH_3 \qquad + \ H_2O$$
$$\qquad\qquad \text{ammonia}$$

Hydrogen is released in many chemical reactions of the bacterial cell. Some cells have the enzymes necessary to combine hydrogen with the nitrates resulting in nitrite and water formation.

In general, it might be said that microorganisms must convert the complex molecules in their medium to simple compounds which can diffuse into their cells. Once inside the cells, the compounds must be changed into usable substances. In order to perform both of these activities, many enzyme systems are necessary. Since not all kinds of bacteria have the same enzyme systems, particular enzymatic reactions can be used as a means of identifying them.

Problem # To study gas production in bacteria.

Background Information

As bacteria use the sugars in broth, they produce acids and gas. The amount of gas produced can be an indication of metabolism. This process of producing gas and acid is called *fermentation*. A special tube, fermentation tube, is used to observe this process.

As bacteria grow and release carbon dioxide, the gas rises through the arm and pushes the level of the broth down. If the fermentation tube is graduated, record the amount of gas formed. This is done by reading the numbers on the graduated side of the tube. If the fermentation tube is not graduated, mark the level of gas formed with a black marking pencil. When the fermentation tube is cleaned, fill it with water. Draw out the water with a pipette until the water level reaches the pencil line. Record the amount of water removed.

Procedure

☐ 1. Fill a sterile fermentation tube with sterile broth.
☐ 2. Flame mouth of culture tube.
☐ 3. Flame wire loop.
☐ 4. Inoculate the fermentation tube.
☐ 5. Flame mouth of fermentation tube and culture tube. Cap both.
☐ 6. At the end of 24 hr. record the amount of gas released. Follow procedure described in the above paragraph. If no acid is formed, no fermentation has occurred.
☐ 7. Complete this chart.

organism	amount of gas
1.	
2.	
3.	
4.	

Questions for Review

1. The amount of gas differs from fermentation tube to fermentation tube. Why?
2. What does fermentation tell us about the growth and number of bacteria?
3. What is the relationship of gas production and the kind of bacteria used in class?

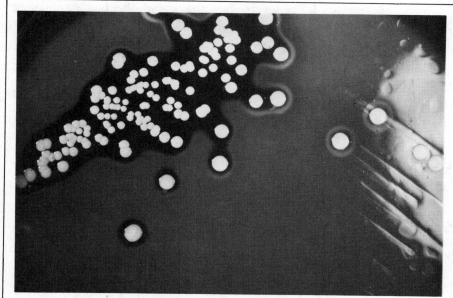

A close up of Staphylococcus colonies on Blood Agar.
Credit: Difco Laboratories

Problem	# To study the enzyme action of bacteria.

Background Information

In the previous exercise, you saw that bacteria can utilize certain sugars for their source of energy. In order to use the sugar, the bacteria had special chemical substances, enzymes, to split out the sugars. There are other kinds of enzymes besides sugar splitting enzymes.

Some bacteria can split starch, others proteins, and others hydrogen peroxide, etc.

Procedure

<u>Peroxide Enzyme — and — Starch Enzyme</u>

☐ 1. Melt a starch agar test tube.
☐ 2. Cool and pour into a Petri dish.
☐ 3. Streak one side of the Petri dish with E. coli. Streak the other side of the Petri dish with B. subtlis.

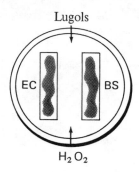

☐ 4. Allow 24 hrs. for growth.
☐ 5. Pour Lugols solution on both streaks at one end of the dish. Do not allow the solution to spread throughout the entire dish.
☐ 6. If the area around the streak turns blue-black, the starch has not been used by the organism (no enzyme). If the area remains unchanged in color, the organism changed the starch to sugar (enzyme present).
☐ 7. Add 2 drops of hydrogen peroxide to the opposite end of the plate.
☐ 8. If bubbling occurs, the organism has the enzyme *catalase*. This changes hydrogen peroxide to water and oxygen (bubbles).

Protein Enzyme

☐ 1. Innoculate 3 nitrate broths with B. subtlis, E. coli, and B. megatherium. Allow the innoculated broth to stand for 24 hours.
☐ 2. Divide the nitrate broth in half
☐ 3. Observe liquification. If the gelatin becomes liquid, the organism has an enzyme which changes the gelatin proteins to amino acids.

Nitrate Enzyme

☐ 1. Inoculate 3 nitrate broths with B. subtlis, E. coli, and B. megatherium.
☐ 2. Divide the nitrate broth in half.
☐ 3. Add 2 drops of NI and 2 drops of NII to one test tube. If a red or pink color appears, the organism can change nitrate to nitrite (reducer). If no color appears, add zinc to the second tube. Add 2 drops of NI and 2 drops of NII several minutes after. If a pink color appears, the organism is a non-reducer (no enzyme).

Question for Review

Organism	Enzyme	Present	Absent
E. coli B. subtlis	starch		
E. coli B. subtlis	catalase		
E. coli B. subtlis	protein	'	
E. coli B. subtlis B. megatherium	nitrate		

1. How can this information be used to identify organisms?

Lesson 17

TEST YOURSELF

Cultural Studies

1. What types of bacteria are motile?
2. What procedure is used to determine motility?
3. The agar tubes in which cultures are maintained are called
4. What name is given to the process that allows colonies to grow in a Petri dish?
5. A substance which speeds up a chemical reaction is called an
6. The process in which energy is released in the absence of oxygen is called
7. The substance on which an enzyme works is called the
8. What enzyme works on hydrogen peroxide?
9. What medium is used to see if bacteria can split proteins?
10. One gas released in fermentation is

1. _____
2. _____
3. _____
4. _____
5. _____
6. _____
7. _____
8. _____
9. _____
10. _____

Answers

1. spirillum
2. hanging drop
3. slants or culture tubes
4. streak plate
5. enzyme
6. fermentation
7. substrate
8. catalase
9. gelatin
10. carbon dioxide or hydrogen

To study the procedures to be followed in identifying an unknown organism.

Lesson 18

Background Information

Every student will be given an organism that is to be identified. Identification is possible only if you know the characteristics of the organism, therefore, you will have to carry out several tests which you have previously learned. Tabulate all results on the summary sheet. To obtain the most accurate results, try to follow the time schedule provided below.

Procedure

Day 1	Make a *simple methylene blue* slide. Examine the slide for the shape and arrangement. Measure the length and width.
Day 2	Make a hanging drop. Determine motility of organism.
Day 3	Make a Gram slide. Determine whether organism is Gram + or -.

Day 4	Transfers
	
	a. Transfer one loopful of the unknown into each nitrate broth.
	
	    brom-cresol milk
	    sugar broths lactose
	                          dextrose
	                          sucrose
	
	b. gelatin stab.
	    sterilize wire needle (straighten out wire loop).
	    flame mouth of culture and gelatin tubes.
	    insert needle into culture tube.
	    stab gelatin ¾ of the way down.
	    flame tubes and cap.
	    place gelatin stab in refrigerator.

Lesson 18

	c. solid media transfers. prepare agar slant. prepare agar plate.
Day 5	Make a spore stain.

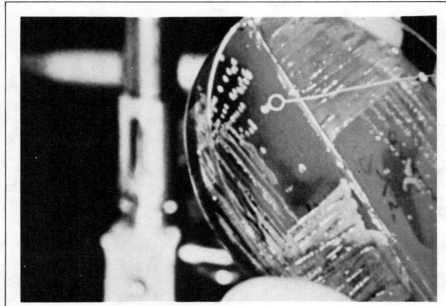

Picking colonies off a primary isolation plate.
Credit: Difco Laboratories

To examine the broths and solid media for identification purposes.

Lesson 19

Background Information

Sugars: Some bacteria use all 3 sugars for growth, others use some of the sugars and still others use none of the sugars.

Procedure

To each fermentation tube add 5 drops of PHENOL RED.
If the broth turns yellow, acid was formed.
If the broth turns red, no acid was formed.
If a bubble is present, in the tube, gas was formed.

Results: Presence of acid and gas
              Presence of acid and no gas   fermentation
              Absence of acid ------------ no fermentation

Gelatin: Some bacteria split gelatin into amino acids.
              When this occurs, the gelatin liquefies.

Results: liquefaction
              no liquefaction

Nitrates: Some bacteria change nitrates to nitrites, others do not.

              Split the contents of the nitrate broth in half. To one half add 2
              drops of each NITRATE I AND NITRATE II. A red color means
              that nitrates were changed to nitrites-NITRATE REDUCER.
              If there is no color, add some grains of ZINC to the second half.
              Wait a few minutes, then add NITRATE I AND II — 2 drops of
              each. A red color means that nitrates were not changed to nitrites
              — non-REDUCER.

Results: REDUCER
              non-REDUCER

Lesson 19

Milk: Some bacteria use the proteins in milk, others do not.

___

If the milk turns purple, it is alkaline (protein used).
If the milk turns yellow, it is acid.

___

Results: Alkaline
          Acid

___

Agar Slant: Determine the color and pattern of colonial growth.
Agar Plate: Determine the color and pattern of colonial growth.

___

BACTERIAL UNKNOWN REPORT

Shape _____ Size _____

Arrangement _____

Motility _____

Gram stain _____

Spores _____

Nitrate _____

Sugar   lactose _____
           dextrose _____
           sucrose _____

Milk _____

Gelatin _____

Agar Slant_____

Agar Plate _____

Vegex (nutrient) broth _____

Compare your test results to those in Bergey's manual and identify your organism.

NAME of Organism _____

Water Analysis

Every living organism needs water for its survival. Man is no exception. However, there are many types of pathogenic organisms which may be transmitted by water. These pathogens cause typhoid fever (Salmonella), cholera (Vibrio), and dysentery (Shigella). Disease-causing organisms gain access to water from fecal waste, indicating that sewage has entered the water.

Today, water pollution is an ever-growing problem. Untreated or improperly treated sewage which may enter drinking water is a health hazard. It is extremely difficult to detect the disease causing organisms in water because they do not occur in great numbers, and they do not live very long in the water. How can we tell if sewage has entered drinking water before an epidemic breaks out?

The water in a *water survey study* is tested for two things, number of bacterial cells present, and the kind of bacteria. Usually water that contains less than 100 cells per 100 ml is considered very good in quality. To make this cell count, a POUR-PLATE technique is used. However, a high bacterial cell count does not necessarily mean that pathogens are present.

Within the intestinal tract of a healthy man there are saprophytic bacteria (Escherichia and Aerobacter). These bacteria are called *coliform* bacteria. Each day billions of these coliforms are normally removed with the feces, therefore, the presence of these organisms in water indicates that sewage is present. Tests designed to detect the coliforms must also be done in a water survey.

Coliform bacteria produce acid and gas in a lactose broth. If a fermentation tube inoculated with a sample of water shows acid and gas, there is a good chance that the coliforms are present. However, other organisms also produce the same reaction. To confirm the presence of coliform bacteria, an EMB (Eosin Methylene Blue) agar plate is streaked with a sample of water.

Escherichia form large, dark almost black colonies with a green-metalic sheen in their centers on EMB. Aerobacter colonies appear as large, pinkish, mucoid colonies with dark centers on EMB. If coliform bacteria are present, the water has been contaminated with sewage and is not drinkable.

To study how to make a Water Survey Analysis.

Problem

Background Information

Every body of water contains countless numbers of microorganisms. To determine the purity of the water, water surveys are made periodically. The water is tested for two things, the number and kinds of bacteria. A special procedure which separates bacterial cells from each other and makes the counting of the colonies easy, is used. This procedure is called a POUR-PLATE.

Procedure

☐ 1. Label 4 test tubes of sterile water 1/10, 1/100, 1/1000, and 1/10,000.
☐ 2. Label 4 Petri dishes 1/10, 1/100, 1/1000, and 1/10,000.
☐ 3. Label the Petri dishes with the name of the place where the water sample was taken.
☐ 4. With a sterile pipette, draw 1 cc of water from the sample.
☐ 5. Discharge pipette into test labeled 1/10.
☐ 6. Tap the sides of the test tube gently to mix contents.
☐ 7. Flame tip of pipette. Remove 1 cc of water from the 1/10 test and discharge into 1/10 Petri dish.
☐ 8. Flame tip of pipette. Remove 1 cc of water from the 1/10 test tube and discharge into 1/100 test tube.
☐ 9. Mix contents by gently tapping sides of test tube.
☐10. Draw 1 cc of water from 1/100 test tube with sterile pipette and discharge into 1/100 Petri dish.
☐11. Flame tip of pipette. Remove 1 cc of water from 1/100 test tube and discharge into 1/1000 test tube.
☐12. Mix contents.
☐13. Flame tip of pipette. Remove 1 cc of water from 1/1000 test tube and discharge into 1/1000 Petri dish.
☐14. Draw 1 cc of water from the 1/1000 test tube with a sterile pipette and discharge into 1/10,000 test tube.
☐15. Flame tip of pipette. Remove 1 cc of water from 1/10,000 test tube and discharge into 1/10,000 Petri dish.
☐16. Cool 4 test tubes of melted agar by rolling between the hand. When the agar is cool enough, pour into each Petri dish.

☐ 17. Gently rotate the Petri dish on the table to mix the water and agar.

☐ 18. Draw 1cc of water from the original sample and discharge into lactose broth fermentation tube.

☐ 19. Prepare an EMB streak plate from original sample.

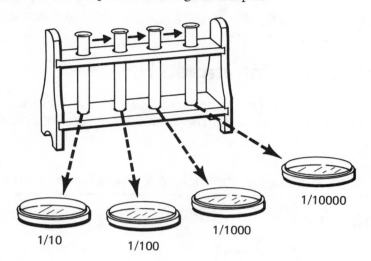

1/10   1/100   1/1000   1/10000

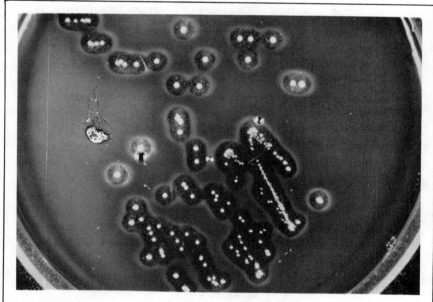

Streptococcus colonies growing on Blood Agar. Notice the clear halos around the colonies. This shows the rupturing of blood cells caused by this organism.
Credit: Difco Laboratories

Problem

To determine the results of the Water Survey Analysis.

Background Information

In order to count the number of colonies in a Petri dish, a colony counter is used. This machine illuminates and magnifies the Petri dish which is placed on a graded plate.

Procedure

☐1. Look at the Petri dishes. Find a dish which shows between 30 and 300 colonies (countable plate).

☐2. Place this dish on the colony counter.

☐3. Count each colony in each square of the plate. Count the colonies which touch the upper and right hand lines of a square as part of that square. Begin the count from left to right.

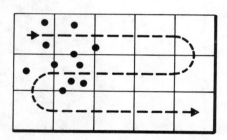

☐4. Record the number of colonies.

☐5. To determine the number of cells per ml. multiply the number of colonies by the dilution of the Petri dish. Ex. 50 colonies are found in the 1/100 dish.

$$50 \times 100 = 5,000 \text{ cells/ml}$$

☐6. Examine the lactose broth. If acid and gas have been formed, there may be coliform bacteria.

☐7. Examine the EMB agar plate.

If large, dark almost black centers with green-metallic sheen colonies appear, Escherichia is present. If large, mucoid, pinkish colonies with dark centers appear, Aerobacter is present. The water is polluted.

Questions for Review

1. Why do you dilute the water samples?
2. Why do you count the plates containing between 30 and 300 colonies?
3. Which water is not drinkable?
4. Does acid and gas in the lactose broth always mean that coliform bacteria are present? Explain.

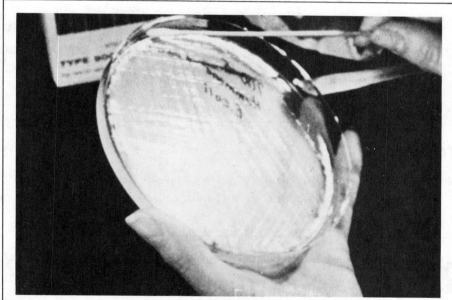

Inoculation of a susceptibility testing plate using a swab dipped into the inoculated broth.
Credit: Difco Laboratories

Problem	# To make a bacterial cell count of milk.

Background Information

Milk is pasteurized before it is sold. Pasteurization kills most disease producing microorganisms (tuberculosis, typhoid fever, diphtheria, scarlet fever, dysentery), but not all of them. It inhibits the growth and reproduction of those which are not killed.

Milk analysis maintains a check on the bacterial cell count. According to the "Milk Ordinance and Code", Grade A pasteurized milk cannot contain more than 200,000/ml (cell count) and not more than 10/ml of coliform bacteria. According to the "Methods and Standards for Production of Certified Milk", pasteurized milk cannot contain more than 10,000/ml and 1/ml of coliforms.

Procedure

☐ 1. Follow the exact procedure for a bacterial cell count of water. The only difference in this procedure is that milk is used instead of a water sample.

Questions for Review

1. Is there any similarity between the diseases resulting from drinking impure milk and water? Explain.
2. What can you say about the relationship of the age of milk and the presence of microorganisms?
3. How do microorganisms get into milk?

To study the effects of disinfectants and antibiotics.

Lesson 23

Background Information

Antibiotics are chemical substances made by living organisms. Antibiotics can destroy or inhibit the growth of bacteria. Penicillin which is produced by a mold is one example of an antibiotic.

Disinfectants are also chemical substances which kill or inhibit the growth of bacteria. Some are more effective than others.

Procedure

- ☐ 1. Divide a Petri dish into 3 equal parts by drawing dividing lines on the bottom of the lower half of the dish.
- ☐ 2. Cool a tube of liquefied agar by rubbing between your hands.
- ☐ 3. Inoculate the agar with 3 loopfuls of an organism.
- ☐ 4. Pour into the Petri dish.
- ☐ 5. Gently rotate Petri dish to mix contents.
- ☐ 6. Pour a disinfectant or antibiotic into a watch glass.
- ☐ 7. Soak small round disks in each substance.
- ☐ 8. Remove a disk with forceps and place in one of the three sections of the Petri dish.
- ☐ 9. Repeat with 2 other disinfectants or antibiotics. Label each section of the dish with a letter or symbol representing the disinfectant.
- ☐10. After 24 hrs., mark a circle around the clear zone around the disk.
- ☐11. Measure the diameter of each clear zone.

If the disinfectant or antibiotic kills the bacteria or prevents their growth, the bacteria will not be found around the disk. The clear area around the disk is called the *zone of inhibition — HALO*. The larger the zone, the more effective is the antibiotic or disinfectant.

Lesson 23

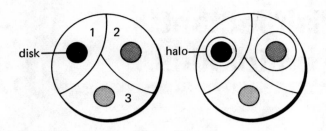

width of zone over

25mm – very effective

20-19 – moderately effective

less than 10mm –slightly effective

Questions for Review

1. What is the difference between an antibiotic and disinfectant.
2. Which are more effective?
3. How do you know which is most effective?

TEST YOURSELF

Applied Bacteriology

1. Bacteria living in the intestinal tract of man are called
2. What microorganisms cause typhoid fever?
3. In what broth do coliforms produce acid and gas?
4. On what solid medium do coliform bacteria grow in a special way?
5. What apparatus helps us count bacterial cells in a water or milk survey?
6. What is the process called which retards or kills bacterial growth in milk?
7. What technique is used to dilute a water sample?
8. Another name for zone of inhibition is
9. In what kind of waste can coliform bacteria be found?
10. A substance extracted from living organisms which kills bacteria is called an

1._____
2._____
3._____
4._____
5._____
6._____
7._____
8._____
9._____
10._____

Answers

1. coliform
2. Salmonella
3. lactose
4. EMB
5. colony counter
6. pasteurization
7. pour plate
8. halo
9. sewage or fecal
10. antibiotic

Glossary

acid-fast   A property of certain bacteria which makes staining them difficult.

agar-agar   A complex sugar extracted from red algae and used to solidify a bacterial medium.

agar slant   A test tube of agar in which the agar is in a slanted position.

antibiotic   A chemical substance obtained from a living organism which kills or inhibits growth of microorganisms.

autoclave   An apparatus using steam under pressure for sterilization.

autotrophic   That which can produce its own food from simple compounds.

broth   A liquid medium.

Brownian movement   A type of movement which is random or haphazard.

coliform   A type of bacteria normally found in the intestinal tract of man.

colony counter   An apparatus used to count the colonies of bacteria.

culture   A population of bacteria grown in a medium.

depression slide   A slide which contains a slight hole in its center.

differential stain   A complex stain used to distinguish between different types of bacteria or different cell structures.

disinfectant   A chemical substance which kills or inhibits the growth of bacteria.

enzyme   A chemical substance which speeds up a chemical reaction.

fermentation   A process in which energy is produced in the absence of oxygen.

fixing   A process which kills and allows bacteria to stick to a slide.

growth curve   A graph that shows the change in the population of bacteria growing in a culture.

heterotrophic   That which cannot produce its own food.

inoculum   The material containing microorganisms which is used for inoculating cultures.

medium   Substance which supports the growth of bacteria.

mordant   A substance which fixes a stain to some part of a bacterial cell.

pathogen   An organism which can cause disease.

Pour Plate   A special technique used to separate cells from each other.

simple stain   A single dye used to color a microorganism.

smear   A thin layer of bacterial material.

spore   A life stage (resting) of bacterial organisms.

stab   A jab of a wire needle containing microorganisms into a medium.

streak plate   A technique used to separate bacterial cells from each other on an agar plate.

vegex   A nutrient broth.

virulence   The ability of an organism to cause disease.

Unit IV

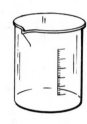

Urinalysis

Unit IV Table of Contents

To The Student

Twenty years ago there was no way to prevent measles. How many measles epidemics occur today?

We live in a scientifically dynamic world where a man can have a second chance at life with a new kidney. Yet, the common problems resulting from infectious disease, genetic defects, and improperly functioning organs remain.

Unfortunately, some day, you may be touched by an illness. Diagnostic tests will be made to determine the cause and extent of your distress. Many of these tests are so common that you hear people talking about them. In this unit, you will learn some simple diagnostic procedures first hand. You will see how these tests are made and learn what the results mean. Knowledge gained through laboratory technology studies have very practical applications in your life.

Who are the technicians who perform these tests? At one time they were students just like you who specialized in laboratory technology. A good technician is a valuable asset to a hospital staff. Who are the people who interpret the results and prescribe and administer the treatment? You may be the doctor or nurse of tomorrow!

There are numerous fields of medical technology to consider and many job opportunities. Perhaps, an introductory course will enable you to see a potential career or encourage you to pursue a medical career. This book and course has been written to assist you to attain your goals. This unit, Urinalysis, has been written to introduce you to the theory and diagnostic tests employed in laboratories. So without further delay, let's begin.

Urinalysis

URINARY SYSTEM

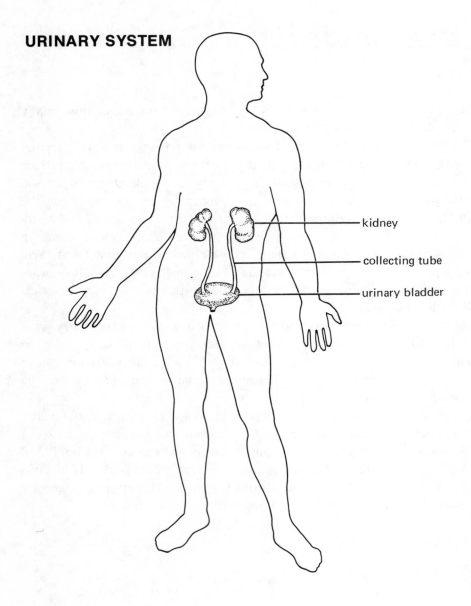

kidney

collecting tube

urinary bladder

Each living cell in the body has the same needs as a single celled organism. As each cell carries out its life activities (metabolism), waste products are formed. These are carbon dioxide, water, soluble salts, and organic matter. Waste products enter the blood stream which transports them to certain organs in the body where they are removed. Water, soluble salts, and organic wastes are filtered out of the blood by the kidneys.

Within each kidney there are approximately one million filtering units, known as *nephrons*. Blood enters the filtering units by way of capillaries which fit into Bowman's capsules, funnel shaped heads of the nephrons. All materials which can pass through the pores of the capillaries leave the blood stream and go into the tubules connected to the capsules. In the tubules reusable materials such as water, some salts and certain proteins are reabsorbed into the blood stream. The waste materials pass from the tubules into a collecting tube which leads to the bladder. The waste material which leaves the tubules and enters the urinary bladder is called *urine*.

NEPHRON

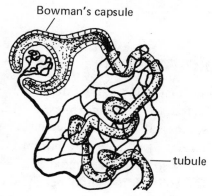

Urine contains water, salts (chlorides, sulfates, and phosphates), and organic wastes (urea, creatinine, and uric acid). The most abundant salt is sodium chloride (NaCl), commonly known as table salt. Urea is the most abundant and most toxic organic waste which comes from the break down of proteins.

Normally, a person excretes 1500 cc of urine per day. The composition of the urine varies from time to time within a given day. The amount of water and other wastes found in the urine depends upon the type of food consumed, the activities engaged in, and the state of health. Below is a chart showing the amount and kind of substances excreted.

Substance	Amount in grams/day
water	1500 grams
chlorides	10-15
phosphates	2.5-3.5
sulfates	1.5-3.0
ammonia	.5-1.0
urea	25-35
uric acid	.4-1

In disease conditions more or less of some of the above substances are found in the urine. More often, there are other substances such as sugar and albumin found in the urine under diseased conditions. Examination of the urine may enable a physician to determine kidney and organic bodily disorders.

Problem   **To study urine collection.**

Background Information

The composition of normal urine varies, depending on the diet and fluid intake. Specimens collected at varying times of the day show different amounts of various substances. If urine is collected 2 or 3 hours after a meal, it will contain large amounts of glucose or albumin. The best time to collect urine is in the early morning so that these molecules will be absent.

Any container used for collection should be chemically clean. Since urine decomposes rapidly, a preservative is sometimes added to the sample. Refrigeration will also reduce decomposition. Urine collected for classroom analysis should be refrigerated until needed.

Procedure

☐ 1. Clean urine bottles. Soak in hot sudsy water, rinse three times. Allow bottle to drip dry.

☐ 2. The first urine passed in the morning is collected in the bottles.

☐ 3. Label the bottle (Name, date).

Questions for Review

1. Why must the bottles used for urine collection be chemically clean?
2. Why is the first urine sample of the morning collected?

To make a physical examination of urine.

Background Information

Urine can be examined without complex tests. This is called a physical examination. This includes color, odor, transparency, sediment, amount, pH, and specific gravity. The last four aspects will be examined in later lessons.

COLOR may be used to detect the presence of abnormal substances in the urine. Usually urine appears almost colorless to amber. The more particles in the urine (higher concentration), the darker it appears. If blood is present, the urine appears red or brown, smoky color. Urine containing bile appears dark orange with a yellow froth when shaken. In cases of diabetes mellitus, the urine appears pale green. Various drugs and foods also give urine an abnormal color which is not an indication of a disease.

ODOR is not a very reliable characteristic to use in detecting diseases. A fruity odor is sometimes associated with diabetes, and a fecal odor might indicate intestinal perforation. In general urine has an aromatic (spicy) odor.

TRANSPARENCY refers to that quality which allows light to pass through. Usually urine is clear. Sometimes it appears cloudy. The cloudiness may be due to several conditions. There may be phosphates present, usually a normal condition. Pus, an indicator of infection, also gives urine a cloudy appearance while blood often gives urine a smoky appearance.

Procedure

☐ 1. Examine the bottle of urine for the above characteristics.
☐ 2. Complete this chart.

Characteristics	Observation
Color	
Odor	
Transparency	

Questions for Review

1. Why is a physical examination important?
2. Why must a physical examination be followed by tests?

Problem
To test the pH of urine.

Background Information

Urine is usually slightly acid. Normal urine ranges from a pH of 4.7 to 8.0. The *average* pH is 6. The pH changes depending on water excretion, emotional stress, tiredness, diet, and the rate of breathing. The urine collected in the morning is less acid than that taken during periods of sleep because the breathing rate is reduced during sleep. The greater the breathing rate, the more acid is the urine. Cereals, meat, and fish make the pH more basic while proteins and fats make the urine more acid. Starvation also makes the urine more acid.

The pH measurement itself merely indicates that there may be an abnormal substance in the urine. It does not tell us what this substance is. Further testing is necessary to determine what abnormal substance is present.

There are many methods for determining pH. You will use several methods and compare the results.

Procedure

☐ 1. NITRAZINE paper - This commercially prepared indicator is accompanied by a color chart. Remove a strip of paper and dip it into a sample of urine. Compare the color of the paper to the chart after one minute.

☐ 2. HYDRION paper - Remove a strip of paper and dip it into a sample of urine. Compare the color of the paper to the chart.

☐ 3. LITMUS paper - Remove a strip of blue litmus paper and dip it into a sample of urine. Observe any color change. Remove a strip of red litmus paper and dip it into a sample of urine. Observe any color change.

☐ 4. Complete this chart.

Indicator	pH
1.	
2.	
3.	

Questions for Review

1. What is pH?
2. Why is pH alone not a good diagnostic tool?

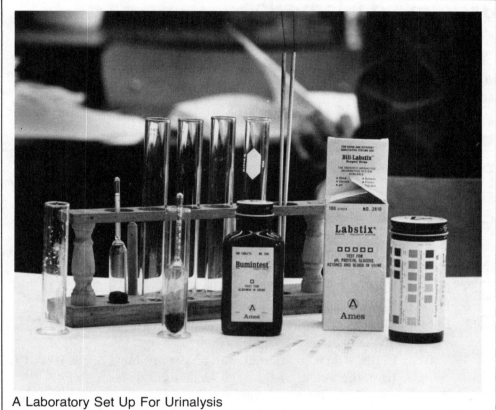

A Laboratory Set Up For Urinalysis

Problem To determine specific gravity.

Background Information

Specific gravity means how many times heavier than water an equal volume of a substance is. By definition the specific gravity of water is 1. The specific gravity of a substance will be less than, equal to, or more than 1, the specific gravity of water.

Procedure

☐ 1. Place a graduate cylinder on a scale and weigh.
☐ 2. Pour 20 ml of alcohol into the cylinder.
☐ 3. Reweigh the cylinder.
☐ 4. Determine the weight of the alcohol by subtracting the weight of the cylinder from the weight of the cylinder and alcohol. Record.
☐ 5. Place another dry graduate cylinder on a scale and weigh.
☐ 6. Place 10 g of salt into the cylinder.
☐ 7. Fill the cylinder with water up to the 20 ml gradation.
☐ 8. Reweigh the cylinder.
☐ 9. Determine the weight of the salt water by subtracting the weight of the cylinder from the weight of the cylinder and salt water. Record.
☐ 10. Place a dry cylinder on a scale and weigh.
☐ 11. Pour 20 ml of water into the cylinder.
☐ 12. Reweigh the cylinder.
☐ 13. Determine the weight of the water by subtracting the weight of the cylinder from the weight of the cylinder and water. Record.
☐ 14. Complete this chart.

Weight of 20 ml	Specific gravity
Water	1
Alcohol	
Salt water	

☐ 15. To determine the specific gravity of alcohol, divide the weight of ordinary water into the weight of alcohol.
☐ 16. To determine the specific gravity of salt water, divide the weight of water into the weight of salt water.

$$S.G. = \frac{Wt\ of\ alcohol}{Wt\ of\ water} \qquad\qquad S.G. = \frac{Wt\ of\ salt\ water}{Wt\ of\ water}$$

Questions for Review

1. Which is heaviest?
2. What is the relationship between the amount of particles in water and its specific gravity?
3. Why is salt water heavier than water?

Problem	# To learn how to use a hydrometer.

Background Informatiom

A special devise, hydrometer, allows you to find the specific gravity of a liquid. The hydrometer consists of a hollow glass tube at the bottom of which is a bulb with a lead shot. The glass tube has gradations. When you place the hydrometer in a liquid, it floats. The level of the liquid also rises. You read the number on the hydrometer which the liquid touches. This gives you the specific gravity of the liquid. The bottom of the meniscus is used in the reading.

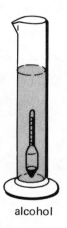
alcohol

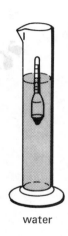
water

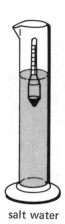
salt water

Procedure

☐ 1. Fill a cylinder with water up to the 0 gradation.
☐ 2. Place the hydrometer into the graduate cylinder. Be sure that the hydrometer does not touch the sides of the cylinder.
☐ 3. Read the number on the hydrometer that the meniscus of the water in the cylinder touches. Record.
☐ 4. Fill a graduate cylinder with alcohol to the 0 gradation.
☐ 5. Place the hydrometer into the cylinder.
☐ 6. Read the meniscus and record.
☐ 7. Fill a graduate cylinder with salt water up to the 0 gradation.

☐ 8. Place the hydrometer into the cylinder.
☐ 9. Read the meniscus and record.
☐ 10. If the hydrometer sinks low, the specific gravity is less than one. If the hydrometer floats high in the cylinder, the specific gravity is greater than one.
☐ 11. Complete this chart.

Substance	Specific Gravity
Alcohol	
Water	1
Salt water	

Questions for Review

1. Draw the hydrometer.
2. What holds the hydrometer up in salt water?
3. What is the effect of the presence of solids in a liquid?
4. How do the results of this lesson compare to the previous lesson?

Problem To determine the specific gravity of urine.

Background Information

Urine is a little heavier than water because it contains solid material such as salt. The normal range of specific gravity is 1.003 to 1.030. The actual value varies within that range depending on diet and the amount of fluid that you drink. In disease conditions, the specific gravity ranges from 1.001 to 1.060. A special hydrometer called a *urinometer* is used to determine the specific gravity of urine.

Procedure

☐ 1. Examine the urinometer. Determine the value of each gradation.

☐ 2. Note a temperature value in the tube of the urinometer. This means that the specific gravity of water = 1 at that temperature.

☐ 3. Check the urinometer to see that it reads 1 at the specific temperature. If it is not off by much, merely subtract this value from the specific gravity of the urine. Ex. If the urinometer reads 1.001 instead of 1.000 in water, subtract .001 from whatever value you obtain when measuring urine.

☐ 4. Fill a cylinder 3/4 full of urine.

☐ 5. Place the urinometer in the cylinder while holding it between the thumb and forefinger.

☐ 6. Spin the urinometer so that it does not touch the sides of the cylinder. If it touches the sides, remove it and start again.

☐ 7. When the urinometer stops spinning, read the bottom of the meniscus. Record the specific gravity.

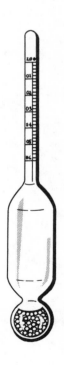

Questions for Review

1. How is the urinometer different from a hydrometer?
2. Why are the values for the specific gravity of urine different for each student?
3. What is the importance of specific gravity to a technician?

Problem

To test for sugar in urine.

Background Information

All cells require energy in order to function. The energy is obtained from the break-down of glucose within the cells. Glucose is brought to the cells by the blood stream which picked it up from the digestive tract. The pancreas produces a hormone, insulin, which in some way makes the cells of the body accept the glucose from the blood stream. If this hormone is absent, the glucose will remain in the blood stream and be excreted by the kidneys. In such a condition, a person will suffer from diabetes mellitus. Urine analysis will, therefore, reveal the presence of sugar in the blood.

Glycosuria or excess sugar in the blood may also occur under normal circumstances. After ingesting a meal rich in carbohydrates, under conditions of stress, anxiety, or fear (examination time), glycosuria occurs. However, in a relatively short time, the blood sugar level will be restored.

Urine analysis is a very important diagnostic tool in the detection of diabetes. A simple test has been devised for the detection of sugar in the urine. In addition to glucose, lactose, levulose, and some pentose sugars may be detected in the urine. However, their presence is not an important diagnostic tool.

Procedure

☐ 1. Pour 5 ml of Benedict's solution into a test tube.
☐ 2. Add 8 to 10 drops of urine to the solution.
☐ 3. Heat to boiling for 2 to 3 minutes.
☐ 4. Allow to cool slowly.
☐ 5. Examine the color and presence of a precipitate.

Color	Amount of Sugar
blue	none
green	trace
greenish-yellow	1%
yellow	less than 2%
orange	2%
brick red	more than 2%

☐ 6. Record.

There are commercially prepared tablets or sticks which can be purchased in a drug store that can be used to detect sugar in the urine. These tablets and sticks are called CLINITEST tablets and CLINITEST sticks.

Procedure

☐ 1. Place 5 drops of urine in a test tube.
☐ 2. Add ten drops of water.
☐ 3. Drop 1 tablet into the test tube. Do not shake tube.
☐ 4. After 15 seconds, shake test tube. Compare the color of the urine in the test tube to the chart.
☐ 5. Record results.

Questions for Review

1. Why are the Clinitest tablets important?
2. Which test is used by a laboratory technician?

Problem To determine the amount of glucose present in the urine.

Background Information

Normal urine may contain 100 to 200 g of sugar over a 24 hour period. The presence of glucose does not necessarily indicate diabetes. Sugar appears in the urine after eating carbohydrates, or may appear under conditions of emotional stress. Sometimes it is important to determine the amount of sugar in the urine. The amount might be used to indicate the stage of the diabetic condition.

Procedure

- [ ] 1. Fill a 50 ml burette with urine.
- [ ] 2. Pipette 25 ml of Benedict solution into a porcelain evaporating dish.
- [ ] 3. Add 7.5 g of sodium carbonate.
- [ ] 4. Heat to boiling and keep mixture boiling. Stir constantly.
- [ ] 5. When the carbonate is dissolved, add urine 2 drops a second until a chalk-white precipitate forms and the blue color begins to fade.
- [ ] 6. Continue to add the urine 2 drops at a time but wait 1/2 minute between additions.
- [ ] 7. You may have to add water to the evaporating dish if the solution gets too thick. If you add water, add a little at a time. Push the precipitate into the solution. Do not allow it to collect on the sides of the dish.
- [ ] 8. When the blue color disappears completely and a yellowish or yellow-green color appears, the experiment is completed.
- [ ] 9. Calculation $\dfrac{50}{c}$ = g per 100 ml of urine

  c = the number of ml from the burette
- [ ] 10. Usually 1500 ml of urine are excreted by an adult daily. You would have to collect the urine over a 24 hour period of time to accurately measure the amount of sugar.
- [ ] 11. Multiply your answer by 15. This gives an inaccurate but acceptable value for the amount of sugar.
- [ ] 12. Record results.

Questions for Review

1. What is one big error in your calculations?
2. If you are examining the urine of a known diabetic, you would dilute it before carrying out the above procedure. Why?
3. Can you give one reason why this test is not often used?

Lesson 9

To test urine for acetone.

Background Information

When the cells of the body cannot burn carbohydrates, other compounds are used. This condition occurs in diabetes and starvation. When fat is used as a source of energy, ketones are produced. This condition is called ketosis. Acetone is a ketone whose presence in the urine usually indicates diabetes.

Procedure

☐1. There are commercially prepared tablets used to detect acetone. Place a tablet on a clean surface—a piece of filter paper.
☐2. Place one drop of urine on the tablet.
☐3. After 30 seconds, compare the color of the tablet with the color chart.

Question for Review

1. What two tests may confirm a diabetic condition?

Problem
To test the urine for diacetic acid.

Background Information

In a diabetic, fats are utilized as a source of energy instead of glucose. The waste products resulting from the break-down of fats are ketones, diacetic acid, and betaoxybutyric acid. Usually, if diacetic acid and ketones are found in the urine, the person has diabetes.

Procedure

☐ 1. Place 5 ml of urine in a clean test tube.
☐ 2. Add ferric chloride a drop at a time until the phosphates precipitate out. Filter the urine.
☐ 3. To the filtered urine, add 2 ml of ferric chloride.
☐ 4. If a red-wine color appears, diacetic acid *may* be present. A further test is necessary to confirm the presence of diacetic acid.
☐ 5. To 5 ml of urine, add 5 ml of distilled water and *one* drop of concentrated nitric acid.
☐ 6. Boil the solution to reduce its volume. Allow to cool and filter if necessary.
☐ 7. If no red-wine color appears, diacetic acid is present.

Question for Review

1. Why is it usually considered positive proof that a person has diabetes if diacetic acid is present?

Diabetes Mellitus

Since the previous group of lessons were useful in detecting diabetes, you should have some understanding of this disorder. A group of cells (Isles of Langerhans) in the pancreas produce a hormone, insulin. No one knows exactly how insulin operates, but it is known that without it, glucose will not be allowed to enter the cells from the blood stream. Therefore, glucose remains in the blood stream and is excreted through the kidneys. The cells in the meantime must obtain energy. They then begin to utilize fats and proteins as a source of energy.

The result of the break-down of fats is a production of ketones. Some ketones leave the body by way of the kidneys. However, if there are too many in the blood to be completely removed, the body attempts to dilute these ketones by removing water from the cells (dehydration). For this reason, a diabetic is usually very thirsty. In addition, the excessive ketones can be smelled on the breath (fruity smell). Eventually, the excessive ketones produce a condition known as acidosis.

Acidosis is a condition in which the pH of the body tissues will change. This means there will be an increase in the hydrogen ion concentration in the body tissues and in the blood stream. A coma which eventually leads to death is the major effect of acidosis on the brain tissue.

Proteins are also utilized for energy. Proteins are essential for the repair of cells. If the proteins are being used, repair is virtually impossible. For this reason the wounds or injuries of a diabetic person do not heal or require a considerable time for healing. This gives bacterial organisms a chance to gain a foothold within the body and, thus, increases the chance of serious infections. In addition, continual use of proteins also results in acidosis.

If diabetes is detected in time, insulin may be administered to prevent the above conditions and to control glucose intake by the cells. In other cases, where the diabetes is not severe, it may be controlled by a simple regulation of the carbohydrate intake or by oral medication.

Problem

To examine the urine for albumin.

Background Information

Certain substances appear in the urine only under pathologic conditions. Proteins are usually present in the urine in amounts so small that they are not detectable. If proteins appear in detectable amounts, this indicates an abnormal condition. One protein not usually found in the urine is albumin (serum albumin). Its presence may indicate a kidney malfunction brought about by certain irritating chemicals (lead, ether, arsenic, mercury, turpentine) or by bacterial toxins (toxins from the diphtheria, scarlet fever, typhoid fever, pneumonia organisms). In addition, albumin in the urine may indicate severe anemia, chronic heart disease, or circulatory disorders.

Procedure

☐ 1. Filter the urine if it is not clear.
☐ 2. Fill a test tube 2/3 of the way with urine.
☐ 3. Heat the upper part of the urine until it begins to boil.
☐ 4. A cloudiness may appear. This may be due to phosphates or to albumin. Add 3 to 5 drops of 10% acetic acid. If the cloud remains and increases, it is due to albumin. If the cloud dissolves, it was due to the phosphates.
☐ 5. The amount of albumin present is recorded with a + sign.
   faint cloudiness +   heavy cloud with no + + +
   heavy cloudiness + +   light passing through a
                          clot of material + + + +
☐ 6. Commercial tablets, BUMINTEST, may also be used. Add 3 tablets to 30 cc of water.
☐ 7. Add equal amount of the solution and urine to a test tube (10 drops of each).
☐ 8. If a cloud appears, albumin is present.

Questions for Review

1. What is the advantage in using the commercial tablets?
2. Why would the acetic acid and heat test be used in a laboratory?

| Problem | **To examine the urine for mucin.** |

Background Information

Mucin is a secretion which appears in the urine when there is an irritation of the mucous membranes of the urinary tract or the vagina. This substance is usually present in small quantities in normal urine. In itself it has no diagnostic value. However, it may be mistaken for albumin and for this reason the urine may be tested for mucin.

Procedure

☐1. Add 6 ml of water to 2 ml of filtered urine.
☐2. Add glacial acetic acid a drop at a time until the urine becomes very acid. If the urine becomes very cloudy, mucin is present.

Questions for Review

1. Why is it important not to confuse mucin with albumin?
2. Why must the urine be filtered before testing for mucin?

TEST YOURSELF

1. What is the normal pH of urine?
2. What is the specific gravity of urine?
3. What chemical can be used in the home to test the urine for sugar?
4. What chemical can be used in the home to test the urine for albumin?
5. What chemical can be used in the home to test the urine for acetone?
6. What is the disease called in which sugar appears in the urine?
7. What substance besides albumin can give urine a cloudy appearance?
8. What substance may appear to be albumin?
9. What are the filtering units in the kidneys called?
10. What type of odor does a diabetic urine have?

1. _____
2. _____
3. _____
4. _____
5. _____
6. _____
7. _____
8. _____
9. _____
10. _____

Answers

1. 6
2. 1.003-1.030
3. Clinitest
4. Bumintest
5. Acetest
6. diabetes
7. phosphates
8. mucin
9. nephrons
10. fruity

Problem # To test the urine for bile.

Background Information

Bile is a complex substance composed of water, bile pigments, bile salts, bile acids, cholesterol, and neutral fats. It is produced in the liver, stored in the gall bladder, and secreted into the small intestine. Here the bile salts and acids serve to emulsify fats so that their digestion may be speeded up. If bile cannot get out of the liver through the bile ducts, it will enter the blood stream. From the blood stream, the bile enters the tissues of the body giving them a yellow coloration. This condition is called jaundice. In addition, the extra bile will leave the blood stream by way of the kidneys and appear in the urine.

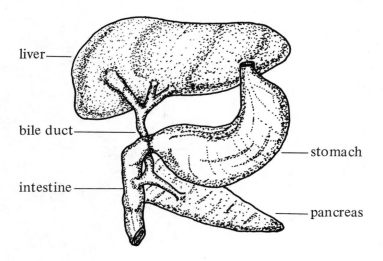

Procedure

☐ 1. Add 5 ml of 10% barium chloride solution to 10 ml of urine. Centrifuge.

☐ 2. Pour off the liquid, and reserve the precipitate. Add 5 ml of water to the precipitate. Mix and filter.

☐ 3. Remove the filter paper which contains the precipitate and place it on a paper towel.

☐ 4. Add 2 drops of Fouchet's Reagent to the precipitate.

☐ 5. If bile is present, a green to blue color will appear.

Laboratory Techniques

Question for Review

1. What is the function of bile?
2. How does bile enter the small intestine?
3. Explain why bile may not be able to enter the small intestine.
4. Why is urine examined for bile?
5. What does the term *jaundice* mean?

Problem	# To examine the urine for urobilinogen.

Background Information

One of the pigments found in bile is biliruben. This pigment is formed when red blood cells are destroyed by the liver. One of the functions of the liver is to remove old worn out red blood cells from the blood stream. The biliruben enters the small intestine and is acted on by bacteria. These organisms convert biliruben to urobilinogen. Several things occur to the urobilinogen.

Some of the urobilinogen is reabsorbed into the blood stream and returned to the liver where it can be recycled. Some of the urobilinogen leaves by way of the large intestine through the feces, and some is excreted through the kidneys. There are several abnormal conditions which interfere with the normal processing of biliruben.

The biliruben may not be able to enter the intestine because of a blockage, therefore, no urobilinogen will be produced. This means that there will be no urobilinogen found in the urine or feces. Secondly, too many red blood cells may be destroyed producing too much biliruben. In this case too much urobilinogen is produced, and it must be removed by the kidneys. This occurs in cases of anemia. Finally, the urobilinogen absorbed into the blood stream from the intestine may not be able to be reabsorbed by the liver. Thus, there will be a high concentration of urobilinogen found in the urine. This condition occurs in cases of hepatitis.

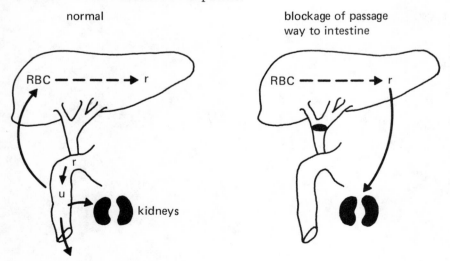

normal   blockage of passage
                          way to intestine

Laboratory Techniques

KEY: RBC - red blood cell
       r   - biliruben
       u - urobilinogen

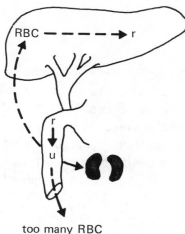

too many RBC
destroyed

urobilinogen not
absorbed by the liver

Procedure

☐ 1. Pipette 10 ml of fresh urine into a test tube.
☐ 2. Add 1 ml of Ehrlich's aldehyde reagent.
☐ 3. If a cherry-red color appears, there is urobilinogen in the urine.

Questions for Review

1. Of what diagnostic value is the test for urobilinogen?
2. Distinguish between the terms biliruben and urobilinogen.

Problem

To test the urine for hemosiderin.

Background Information

When there is excessive destruction of red blood cells, hemoglobin is released into the blood stream. The hemoglobin is broken down by cells in the kidneys. One of the components of this break-down is an iron compound, hemosiderin. Destruction of red blood cells results in a condition called anemia. The hemosiderin test coupled with blood analysis gives evidence of the presence of anemia. Further blood tests would have to be performed to determine the cause of anemia.

Procedure

☐ 1. Centrifuge 15 ml of fresh urine.
☐ 2. With a micropipette, remove the liquid after centrifuging.
☐ 3. Place some of the sediment on a slide and examine. If there are brown granules in the epithelial cells, hemosiderin may be present.
☐ 4. To the rest of the sediment, add 2 ml of potassium ferrocyanide solution and 2 ml of hydrochloric acid. Mix well.
☐ 5. Allow to stand for 10 minutes. Centrifuge and remove liquid.
☐ 6. Examine the sediment for the presence of blue granules. The blue granules confirm the presence of hemosiderin.

Questions for Review

1. How is blood and urine analysis combined to diagnose disease?
2. Why will the granules be found in epithelial cells of the kidney?
3. What blood tests would confirm anemia?

To test the urine for homogentisic acid.

Background Information

Proteins are composed of amino acids. When the proteins are digested, the amino acids are released. The amino acids are then converted into the vital substances that the body needs. One disease which arises because of defective amino acid conversion is PKU, phenylketonuria.

Phenylalanine (an amino acid) is normally converted to tyrosine. Tyrosine in turn may be changed to melanin, the pigment of skin and hair. Sometimes phenylalanine is not changed to tyrosine. It remains in the blood stream and damages the brain cells. A child born with this defect will become mentally retarded. Homogentisic acid is usually found in the urine of an individual who has PKU. In addition the urine is colored brown to black. Today, the urine of all new born infants is tested to make sure that this defect is absent. If a child is born with PKU, a special diet will control the condition permitting the child to develop normally.

Procedure

☐ 1. Place 5 ml of urine in a test tube.
☐ 2. Add a few drops of ferric chloride solution a drop at a time.
☐ 3. If an unstable green to blue color appears, homogentisic acid is present.

Questions for Review

1. Why is the test for PKU important?
2. How can a doctor find out if an infant has PKU?

To examine the urine microscopically for sediment.

17

Background Information

Normal urine contains solid particles, sediment. The sediment is composed of various solids, crystals, cells, casts, fats, mucous threads, bacteria, and spermatozoa. The presence of any of these particles is not diagnostic of a disease. The type of solid in the sediment and its abundance may be used as a diagnostic tool. For example, if red blood cells are found free in the urine, or combined with casts, this is indicative of a renal disorder. Below are pictures of a few types of solids that may be found in the urine.

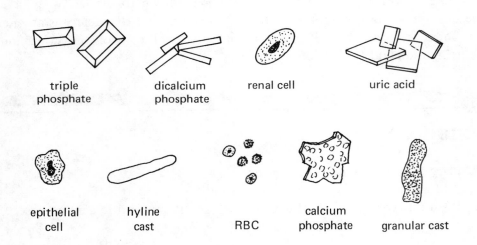

triple phosphate   dicalcium phosphate   renal cell   uric acid

epithelial cell   hyline cast   RBC   calcium phosphate   granular cast

Procedure

☐ 1. Obtain a fresh sample of urine.
☐ 2. Pipette 15 ml into a centrifuge tube.
☐ 3. Centrifuge for 3 to 5 minutes.
☐ 4. Pipette most of the clear fluid off and discard it.
☐ 5. Pipette one drop of sediment on to a clean slide.

☐ 6. Cover with a cover slip.

☐ 7. Examine under LP – reduce the light by closing the diaphragm. The casts should appear as "ghosts" against a dark background.

☐ 8. Switch to HP to examine the casts or other particles in closer detail. Open the diaphragm.

☐ 9. Draw each type of sediment that you find in the urine.

Questions for Review

1. If normal urine contains casts, how can their presence be used to diagnose a disease?

2. Is there any relationship between the cloudiness of the urine and the amount and type of sediment found?

To determine the amount of sediment present in the urine.

Background Information

Casts are impressions of the tubules of the nephrons in the kidneys. Albumin often sticks to the walls of the tubules forming an impression of the walls. Eventually, the casts are washed off the walls and appear in the urine. As the casts come off the walls, they will remove materials that were imbedded in the walls. Abnormal particles (RBC) that were imbedded in the walls of the tubules will be drawn along with the casts. By examining the casts, an abnormal substance can be detected. The number of casts and the type of casts may reveal a kidney disorder. An overabundance of one particular kind of cell may also indicate a disorder.

Procedure

☐ 1. The urine sample should be the first urine voided in the morning. How many hours passed from the last voiding to the taking of the urine samples?

☐ 2. Calculation

$$\frac{\text{amount of urine collected}}{\text{number of hours x 5}} = \begin{array}{l}\text{volume of urine} \\ \text{used for test}\end{array}$$

☐ 3. Place the amount calculated into a graduate centrifuge tube and centrifuge for 2 - 3 minutes.

☐ 4. Remove the liquid up to the .5 ml gradation in the centrifuge tube.

☐ 5. Mix the sediment in the tube.

☐ 6. With a pipette place one drop of sediment in a blood counting chamber.

☐ 7. Place the counting chamber on the microscope and reduce the light.

☐ 8. Count the casts in the ruled area.

☐ 9. Count the number of cells in the ruled areas.

Laboratory Techniques

☐10. Complete this chart.

Count			Total
No. of casts	x	100,000	
No. of cells	x	1,000,000	

sum

☐11. Acceptable counts range from 400,000-500,000 for RBC, 1,000,000 WBC and epithelial cells, 5,000 casts.

Questions for Review

1. Why is the urine centrifuged first?
2. Why do you mix the sediment after most of the fluid is removed?
3. Why is fresh urine most useful in searching for casts?
4. What objective of the microscope do we use in this procedure?
5. Why is urine examined for casts?

Problem To determine the amount of urea in the urine.

Background Information

Urea is made in the liver from the break-down of proteins. It is excreted into the blood stream and removed by the kidneys. Normal urine contains 15 to 35 mg of urea. This is the amount that would be excreted over a period of 24 hours. To determine the amount of urea in the urine, two procedures are involved. One procedure changes urea to ammonia and the other measures the amount of ammonia (titration).

Urease is an enzyme which changes urea into ammonia. The urease works best in a buffered (neutral) solution. The ammonia set free in tube A travels to B where it combines with the acid, neutralizing the acid. If some of the ammonia does not mix with the acid, it enters tube C where it is trapped in the undiluted urine. K_2CO_3 sets it free again. The ammonia set free enters tube D and neutralizes the acid. In order to find out how much ammonia was released from the urine, titration is carried out.

Procedure

☐ 1. Add 25 ml of 4% boric acid to tube B and D. Add .7 ml of brom-cresol green solution, 1 drop of caprylic alcohol to tube B and D. Stopper but do not connect.

☐ 2. Dilute 5 ml of urine to 50 ml. Add 3 ml of diluted urine, 3 ml of buffer solution, 2 drops of caprylic alcohol, .5 ml of urease solution into tube A. Stopper but do not connect. Clamp rubber tubes. Allow to stand 15 to 20 minutes.

☐ 3. Add 2 drops of alcohol to 5 ml of 5% sulfuric acid into tube W.

☐ 4. Attach tubes C and D and begin suction. While the air current is running, add 10 ml of K_2CO_3 saturated solution into tube C and pipette 3 ml of undiluted urine through the inlet tube.

☐ 5. Connect tube A, B, and C.

☐ 6. Run air current slowly for 2 minutes, then speed up.

☐ 7. Run air for 20 minutes.

☐8. Decrease air flow and disconnect middle tubes first. The tubes closest to the suction are disconnected last.

☐9. Titrate. (The next lesson provides the procedure for titration.)

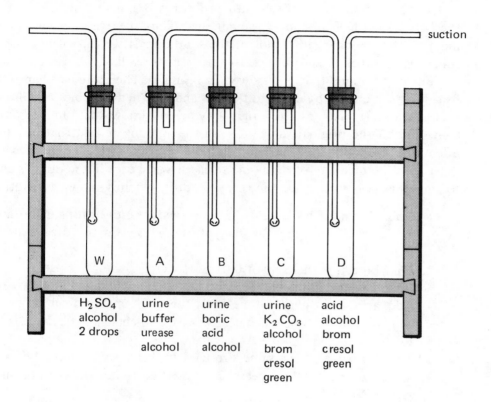

W	A	B	C	D
H_2SO_4 alcohol 2 drops	urine buffer urease alcohol	urine boric acid alcohol	urine K_2CO_3 alcohol brom cresol green	acid alcohol brom cresol green

suction

Questions for Review

1. What is urea?
2. What is the relationship between
   a) urea and the liver
   b) urea and the kidneys
3. How much urea is contained in normal urine?
4. What is the difference between urea and urease?

Procedure - Titration

BACKGROUND INFORMATION

The base, ammonia, diffuses into test tubes B and D. The acid content of these tubes is decreased by the ammonia. Thus there is a change of pH as indicated by the change in color of the solutions. If we can change the pH of solutions in tubes B and D back to the original reading, we can compute the amount of ammonia that is dissolved in B and D. Therefore we change the pH by adding acid, drop by drop, to tubes B and D. When the color of solutions in tubes B and D matches the original, you will know that the pH has been converted to the original value. Record the amount of acid that you used to effect the color change. The amount of acid used in the titration will help determine the quantity of ammonia released when urea in the urine is changed to ammonia. A burette is used in this procedure which is known as titration.

1. Place 25 ml of boric acid, 25 ml of water, and 2 drops of brom-cresol green in a test tube the size of those used in the urea experiment-CONTROL.
2. Fill a burette with 25 ml of 0.01 N H_2SO_4.
3. Place test tube B under the burette.
4. Add acid a drop at a time until the color matches the color of the control. Record how much acid was used to change the color.
5. Record _____ ml = A_1.
6. To a test tube of the same size used in this lesson, add 3 ml of water, 3 ml of buffer, .5 ml of urease, 2 drops of alcohol, 2 drops of brom-cresol green-CONTROL.
7. Titrate tube A until the color matches.
8. Record the amount of acid used to match the colors.
9. Record _____ ml = C_1.
10. Subtract A_1 - C_1 and multiply by 50. This gives you the number of mg. of nitrogen released from urea and ammonia in 100 ml of urine.
11. Add 25 ml of boric acid, 2 drops of alcohol, 2 drops of brom-cresol green to a test tube-CONTROL.
12. Titrate tube D. Record ml of acid = A_2.
13. Add 3 ml of water, 10 ml of K_2CO_3, 2 drops of alcohol, and 2 drops of brom-cresol green-CONTROL.
14. Titrate tube C. Record ml of acid = C_2.
15. Subtract A_2 - C_2 and multiply by 5. This gives us the number of mg of nitrogen ammonia per 100 ml of urine.
16. Final calculation: Subtract the answer from step 15 from step 10's answer.

$$50 (A_1 - C_1) - 5 (A_2 - C_2) = \text{amount of urea}$$

Questions for Review

1. Is the calculated amount of urea normal in your urine sample?
2. What are some of the sources of error in your calculations?

TEST YOURSELF

1. Where is bile produced?
2. What do you call the condition in which bile is present in the body tissues?
3. What machine is used to separate solid particles from liquids?
4. What is an abnormal bile pigment found in the urine?
5. What pigment may be found in the urine of an anemic person?
6. What amino acid can cause mental retardation?
7. What do you call the disease that results in a mentally retarded child?
8. What do you call the impressions of the kidney tubules?
9. What do you call the toxic nitrogen compound excreted by the kidneys?
10. What do you call the process of neutralizing a base by slowly adding an acid?

1. _____
2. _____
3. _____
4. _____
5. _____
6. _____
7. _____
8. _____
9. _____
10. _____

Answers

1. liver
2. jaundice
3. centrifuge
4. urobilinogen
5. hemosiderin
6. phenylalanine
7. phenylketonuria
8. casts
9. urea
10. titration

Urine Analysis Summary Sheet

NORMAL URINE SAMPLE

Physical examination
     color _____
     odor _____
     transparency _____
pH _____
Specific Gravity _____
Sugar _____
Acetone _____
Diacetic Acid _____
Albumin _____
Mucin _____
Bile _____
Hemosiderin _____
Homogentisic Acid _____
Type of Casts _____
Type of Cells _____
Number of casts _____
Number of cells _____

UNKNOWN URINE SAMPLE

Physical examination
     color _____
     odor _____
     transparency _____
pH _____
Specific Gravity _____
Sugar _____
Acetone _____
Albumin _____
Bile _____
Urobilinogen _____

Glossary

acetest   Commercial tablets used to detect ketones in the urine.

albumin   A protein not usually found in the urine.

bile   A secretion made in the liver which emulsifies fats in the small intestine.

bumintest   Commercial tablets used to detect albumin in the urine.

casts   Impressions of the tubules of the nephrons.

clinitest   Commercial tablets used to detect sugar in the urine.

diabetes   A disease caused by the lack of insulin.

hydrometer   A device used to measure specific gravity.

insulin   Hormone that regulates blood sugar.

ketone   A chemical which is produced from the break-down of fats.

mucin   A secretion of the urinary tract that is found in the urine.

nephron   A filtering unit in the kidney.

pH   Measure of the hydrogen ion concentration.

phenylketonuria   A disorder in which phenylalanine cannot be changed to tyrosine.

protein   A complex chemical substance.

specific gravity   The measure of the heaviness of a substance compared to water.

urea   A toxic chemical substance which comes from the break-down of nitrogen containing compounds.

urinometer   Device that measures the specific gravity of urine.

Appendix

METRIC CONVERSION TABLES OF LENGTH

METRIC SYSTEM	ENGLISH SYSTEM
Abbreviations:	in = inch
mm = millimeters	ft = foot
cm = centimeters	yd = yard
m = meter	mi = mile

METRIC UNITS OF LENGTH	ENGLISH EQUIVALENTS
10 mm = 1 cm	2.5 cm = 1 in.
100 cm = 1 m	25 mm = 1 in.
1000 m = 1 km	1 m = 39 in.

HOW TO CONVERT FROM THE ENGLISH SYSTEM TO THE METRIC SYSTEM IN LENGTH

When you know		*multiply by*		*to find*	
	inches		2.5		centimeters
	feet		30		centimeters
	yards		0.9		meters
	miles		1.6		kilometers

METRIC CONVERSION TABLES OF VOLUME

METRIC SYSTEM	ENGLISH SYSTEM
Abbreviations:	tsp = teaspoons
ml = milliliters	Tbsp = tablespoons
cc = cubic centimeters	fl oz = fluid ounce
l = liters	pt = pints
	qt = quarts
	gal = gallons

METRIC UNITS OF VOLUME	ENGLISH EQUIVALENTS
1000 ml = 1.0 *l* (liter) *	29.5 cc = 1 fl oz.
1 ml = 1 cc	1.0 *l* = 1.06 qt.
	29.5 ml = 1 fl oz.

*The abbreviation for *liter* is the small letter *l*. Care must be taken that the letter *l* is not confused with the number "1".

HOW TO CONVERT FROM THE ENGLISH SYSTEM
TO THE METRIC SYSTEM IN VOLUME

When you know		multiply by		to find	
When you know	teaspoons	multiply by	5	to find	milliliters
	tablespoons		15		milliliters
	fluid ounces		30		milliliters
	cups		0.24		liters
	pints		0.47		liters
	quarts		0.95		liters
	gallons		3.8		liters

METRIC CONVERSION TABLES OF WEIGHT (MASS)

METRIC SYSTEM

Abbreviations:

mg = milligrams
g = grams
kg = kilograms
t = tonnes

ENGLISH SYSTEM

oz = ounces
lb = pounds

METRIC UNITS OF WEIGHT

1000 mg = 1 g
1000 g = 1 kg

ENGLISH EQUIVALENTS

28.3 g = 1 oz.
453.6 g = 1 lb.
0.45 kg = 1 lb.

HOW TO CONVERT FROM THE ENGLISH SYSTEM
TO THE METRIC SYSTEM IN WEIGHT (MASS)

When you know		multiply by		to find	
When you know	ounces	multiply by	28	to find	grams
	pounds		0.45		kilograms
	{ short tons 2000 lb		0.9		tonnes

PREFIXES USED IN THE METRIC SYSTEM

Greek Prefixes Indicating MORE Than the Unit	UNIT	Latin Prefixes Indicating A PART of the Unit
Kilo = 1000	LITER	Deci = 0.1 (one tenth)
Hecto = 100	METER	Centi = 0.01 (one hundredth)
Deca = 10	GRAM	Milli = 0.001 (one thousandth)

TEMPERATURE CONVERSIONS

When you know	Fahrenheit	*multiply by*	5/9 (after subtracting 32)	*to find*	Celsius
	Celsius		9/5 (then add 32)		Fahrenheit

Glossary

ABO system   A system of classifying or typing blood.

Acid-fast   A property of certain bacteria which makes staining them difficult.

agar-agar   A complex, jelly-like substance extracted from red algae and used to solidify a bacterial medium.

agar slant   A test tube of agar in which the agar is in a slanted position.

agglutinin   A protein found in red blood cells.

agglutinogen   A protein found in blood plasma.

albumin   A protein found normally in the blood and in serous fluids, but not usually present in urine.

amoeboid   Having the shape and movement of an amoeba.

analytical balance   A sensitive scale that is accurate to 0.0001 g.

antibody   A chemical substance (protein) produced by the body to combat antigens.

antibiotic   A substance produced by soil molds or other living organisms which is toxic to individuals of other species.

antigen   A protein foreign to body tissues which stimulates the formation of antibodies.

autoclave   An apparatus using steam under pressure for sterilization.

autotrophic   An organism that can produce its own food by utilizing in-organic materials.

bile   A secretion made in the liver which emulsifies fats in the small intestine.

broth   A liquid medium in which bacteria are grown.

Brownian movement   A movement of molecules or particles which is random or haphazard.

bumintest   Commercial tablets used to detect albumin in the urine.

bunsen burner   A burner which produces a high temperature without soot.

casts   Impressions of kidney tubules.

centimeter   A measure of length.

chromatography   A technique used to separate closely related chemical substances.

clinitest   Commercial tablets used to detect sugar in the urine.

colony counter   A piece of equipment used to count bacterial colonies.

coliform   A species of bacteria normally found in the intestinal tract of man.

compound microscope   A light microscope having a double lens system.

culture   A population of bacteria grown in or on a medium.

depression slide   A microscope slide that has a well or depression in the center.

diabetes   A disease caused by the lack of insulin resulting in the inability of cells to utilize sugar.

dial-o-gram   A scale with a vernier mechanism that weighs accurately to 0.01 g.

differential count   A counting of the different types of white blood cells on a stained smear.

differential stain   A complex stain used to distinguidh between different types of bacteria or various cell structures.

disinfectant   A fluid that is used to kill or inhibit the growth of bacteria.

electrode   Either of the two poles of a battery that can send out or detect small electrical charges.

enzyme   A protein molecule that speeds up a chemical reaction.

fermentation   A respiratory process in which energy is produced in an environment of decreased oxygen.

flanging   A process of strengthening the edges of glassware.

fire polishing   A process of smoothing the edges of rough glassware by melting in a flame.

fixing   A process which kills bacteria and allows them to stick to the slide.

graduate   A piece of glassware in which known gradations are etched into its side.

growth curve   A graph that shows the change in the population of bacteria that are growing in a culture.

Hayems solution   A fluid used to destroy white blood cells and to dilute red blood cells for counting.

hemacytometer   A ruled slide or counting chamber used in making blood counts.

hemoglobin   A red pigment in red blood cells which serves as an oxygen carrier.

heterotroph   An organism that cannot produce its own food from inorganic materials.

hydrometer   A device used to measure specific gravity.

indicator   A chemical that detects the presence of hydrogen ions or hydroxyl ions.

inoculum   Microorganisms that are used for inoculating cultures.

insulin   A hormone that regulates blood sugar.

ketone   A chemical which is produced by the breakdown of fats.

lancet   A pointed instrument that is used to make a finger puncture.

leukocyte   Another name for a white blood cell.

liter   A measure of volume.

medium   A liquid or solid material that supports the growth of bacteria.

meter   A measure of length.

metric system   A system used in scientific measurements.

micrometer, ocular   A ruled scale in the ocular (eyepiece) of a microscope.

micrometer, stage   A ruled scale on a slide used to calibrate the ocular micrometer

micron   A measure of length used in microscopic work. One micron is equal to 0.001 of a mm.

milliliter   A measure of volume, 0.001 of a liter.

millimeter   A measure of length, 0.001 of a meter.

mordant   A chemical that fixes a stain to some part of a bacterial cell.

mucin   A secretion of the urinary tract that is found in the urine.

nephron   A filtering unit in the kidney.

Oil immersion   A microscope lens that can be immersed in oil.

pathogen   An organism which can cause disease.

percentage solution   A solution in which the concentration is measured on the basis of 100 ml.

pH   A measure of the hydrogen ion concentration of a solution.

pH meter   A piece of equipment (a meter) used to measure the pH of a solution.

phagocytic   Having the ability to ingest microorganisms.

phenylketonuria   A disorder in which phenylalanine cannot be metabolized to tyrosine.

pipette   A graduated glass measuring tube used to transfer or measure specific amounts of liquids.

plasma   The liquid part of the blood.

platelet   A type of blood cell necessary for blood clotting.

pour plate   A special technique used to separate cells from each other.

protein   A complex chemical substance; an organic molecule.

serum   The liquid part of the blood which is free from fibrinogen.

simple stain   A single dye used to color a microorganism.

smear   A thin layer of bacterial material.

solute   Particles that are dissolved in a solution.

solution   The result of dissolving a solute in a solvent.

solvent   A dissolving agent for a solute.

specific gravity   The measure of the heaviness of a chemical substance compared to water.

spore   The resting stage of a bacterium.

stab   A jab of wire needle into an agar butt. The needle is usually inoculated with bacteria.

stain   A dye that is used to color cells and cell parts.

streak plate   A technique used to separate bacterial cells from each other on an agar plate.

thermometer   A device for the measurement of temperature.

Thoma pipette   A pipette used for diluting blood.

triple beam balance   A scale which weighs accurate to 0.1 g.

urea   A protein compound that comes from the breakdown of nitrogen-containing materials.

urinometer   A device that measures the specific gravity of urine.

vegex   A commercial nutrient broth.

virulence   The ability of an organism to cause disease.

volume   The capacity of a container.

Wright's stain   A stain used to distinguish the different types of blood cells by giving them color.

Bibliography

Best, C.H. and N.B. Taylor. THE HUMAN BODY — ITS ANATOMY AND PHYSIOLOGY. 4th ed. Holt, Rinehart and Winston, New York, 1963.

BIOLOGY HANDBOOK. Bureau of Secondary Curriculum Development, The New York State Education Department, Albany, 1960.

Bleifeld, M. MODERN BIOLOGY IN REVIEW. Barron's Educational Series, Inc. N.Y., 1972.

Conn, H.J. BIOLOGICAL STAINS. 7th ed. Williams and Wilkins Co., Baltimore, 1965.

Diggs, L.W. et al. THE MORPHOLOGY OF BLOOD CELLS IN WRIGHT STAINED SMEARS OF PERIPHERAL BLOOD AND BONE MARROW. Abbot Laboratories Monograph, Chicago, 1954.

Davidsohn, I. and B. Wells. CLINICAL DIAGNOSIS BY LABORATORY METHODS. W.B. Saunders Co., Phila., 1966.

Edwards, G. BIOLOGY INTRODUCTION TO LIFE — LABORATORY MANUAL. Addison Wesley Co., Menlo Park, 1969.

Frobisher, M. FUNDAMENTALS OF MICROBIOLOGY. W.B. Saunders Co., Phila., 1968.

Guyton, A.C. FUNDAMENTALS OF THE HUMAN BODY. W.B. Saunders Co., Phila., 1964.

HEALTH CAREERS (Auxiliary Health Ass't - 11th and 1th years). Curriculum Bulletin 12B, Board of Education, City of New York, 1964-65.

LABORATORY PROCEDURES IN CLINICAL BACTERIOLOGY. Department of the Army, TM 8-227-5, Gov't Printing Office, Washington, 1963.

LABORATORY PROCEDURES IN CLINICAL CHEMISTRY AND URINALYSIS. Dept. of the Air Force, AFM 160-49, Gov't Printing Office, Washington, 1967.

LABORATORY PROCEDURES IN CLINICAL HEMATOLOGY. Department of the Army, TM 8-227-4, Gov't Printing Office, Washington, 1963.

Lyne, E. and R.O. Capella. LABORATORY EXERCISES IN MICROBIOLOGY. Dept. of Science and Mathematics Education, New York University, New York, 1968.

METHODS FOR MEDICAL LABORATORY TECHNICIANS. Dept. of the Army and Air Force, TM 8-227, AFM 160-14, Gov't Printing Office, Washington, 1951.

Morholt, E. et al. A SOURCEBOOK FOR THE BIOLOGICAL SCIENCES. 2nd ed., Harcourt, Brace and World, N.Y., 1966.

Pelczar, M.J. MICROBIOLOGY. McGraw Hill, New York, 1965.

Rogers, C.L. ESSENTIALS OF BIOLOGY—A Basic Text of Current Biological Thought. Barron's Educational Series, Inc., N.Y., 1967.

Ruch, T.C. and J.F. Fulton. MEDICAL PHYSIOLOGY AND BIO-PHYSICS. 18th ed., Saunders, Co., Phila., 1960.

Stehli, G. THE MICROSCOPE AND HOW TO USE IT. Sterling Publ., New York, 1968.

Youmans, W.B. HUMAN PHYSIOLOGY. Revised ed., Macmillan, New York, 1962.

Weisz, P.B. THE SCIENCE OF BIOLOGY. McGraw-Hill, New York, 1963.

NOTES

NOTES

NOTES